ARTHRITIS

O P T I M A

ANSWERS TO
ARTHRITIS

TONY VAN DEN BERGH

ILLUSTRATED BY ANDRE YANIW

An OPTIMA book

© Tony van den Bergh 1987

First published in 1987 by
Macdonald Optima, a division of
Macdonald & Co. (Publishers) Ltd

A BPCC PLC company

BRITISH LIBRARY CATALOGUING IN PUBLICATION DATA
Van den Bergh, Tony
    Arthritis..—(Healthlines).
    1. Arthritis—Diet therapy
    I. Title   II. Series
    616.7'2206   RC933

    ISBN 0-356-12436-3

Macdonald & Co. (Publishers) Ltd
3rd Floor
Greater London House
Hampstead Road
London NW1 7QX

Photoset in 11/13pt Century by
🅐 Tek Art Limited, Croydon, Surrey

Made and printed in Great Britain by
The Guernsey Press Co. Ltd., Guernsey, Channel Islands.

To Annette Spence without whose help this book would never have been written.

Thanks to:
Richard Rushman FRCS for his surgical skill which restored my mobility and ended my pain; Anne Beaugié for the spinal anaesthetic which enabled me to remain conscious throughout my hip replacement, so I could see what was being done; Gail Darlington, consultant physician, for her research on diet and arthritis; Sheila Lee for her information on thalassotherapie; Alan Dixon FRCS for permission to lift some of his words; Laura Mitchell for advice on relaxation and coping in the home; Jenny Reason of the Royal Free Hospital for details of occupational therapy aids and Annette Spence SRN, psycho-sexual counsellor of the Marie Stopes Clinic, for her information on sex and arthritis.

CONTENTS

1.
WHAT IS ARTHRITIS?

ARTHRITIS IS . . .

Arthritis is a condition of the body's joints. Well over half of us will suffer from it at some time in our lives, usually in our later years. The word 'arthritis' is used to describe many different conditions in which the only common factor is pain in the joints. The pain, however, can vary from mild twinges to an agony so intense and so damaging that the sufferer can become totally housebound.

Strictly speaking, 'arthritis', which comes from the Greek word for bone, means 'inflammation of the joint', although in osteoarthritis, which is more to do with wear and tear, inflammation plays little part. 'Arthrosis' is the term the medical profession use to describe such conditions, although most of the rest of us use 'arthritis' indiscriminately.

Our bodies have two major types of joint: the hinge and the ball and socket. A hinge joint, for instance the elbow, facilitates one simple, direct, up and down movement. A ball and socket joint, such as the hip, combines the up and down movement with rotation – a much more complicated procedure. As well as facilitating movement, joints provide stability, without which we

9

would be like raggety dolls, lurching about with every movement.

Arthritis can affect most but not all of our joints. There are, for instance, joints in our skulls, which during birth allow the skull to narrow and so pass more easily through our mother's birth canal. Then they fuse and become, in effect, solid bone and so are impervious to arthritic disease. There are also other joints, of a cartilaginous

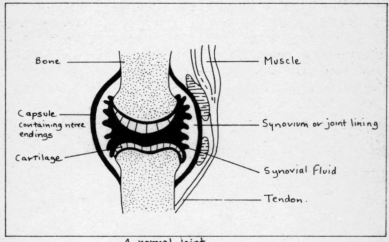

A normal joint.

nature, which only move at specific times and which, when not in use, are immobile and so safe. For example the joint in the front of a woman's pelvic girdle only moves when she is giving birth, when it allows the canal through which her child is born to widen.

The joints most at risk from arthritis are the synovial joints. In these joints the ends of the bones are covered by cartilage (a pearly gristle), encased in a membrane and lubricated by the synovial fluid. This lubrication is most important for any joint because without it the bones of the joint would quickly erode, or wear away.

Over 20 million people in Britain suffer from arthritis, and over eight million have it sufficiently severely to seek medical advice each year. The expense to the country is enormous. Over eight million working days are lost annually at a cost of over £1,000 million. Almost one third of all patients seen by doctors have some form of rheumatism which, although medically-speaking is an ill-defined term, does include all types of arthritis. And the situation is similar throughout most of the developed world.

The cost in human suffering is, however, far greater than any statistics can possibly indicate. Arthritis can be both extremely painful and crippling. Going out of the house, let alone working, can become impossible. Ordinary everyday activities, which most of us do without thinking, like getting on buses or in and out of cars, making tea or using the lavatory, become labours to daunt Hercules. Arthritis can completely destroy that most precious individual right – independence.

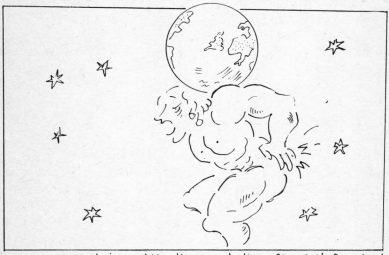

One more twinge like that and they can get somebody else to carry their blooming planet.

THE DIFFERENT TYPES OF ARTHRITIS

Osteoarthritis
Osteoarthritis is the most common arthritic condition and affects 50 per cent of all adults in Britain at some

time in their lives. In any one year over five million people will be receiving treatment for it in some form or other. Men and women are affected equally, but with one major difference: in women it is common to find several damaged joints rather than one, which is the common pattern among men.

It is a degenerative condition involving the disintegration of the cartilage of the affected joint and, unlike rheumatoid arthritis, it does not usually cause

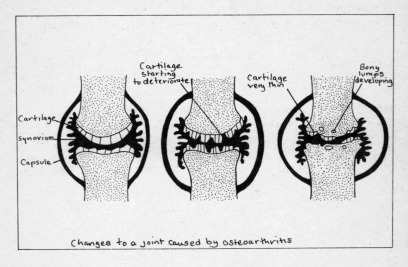

Changes to a joint caused by osteoarthritis

any constitutional disturbance. It can, however, dramatically distort the personality of someone suffering from it as constant pain and the frustration of limited movement can make them irritable and often irrational.

Osteoarthritis is unknown in childhood and rare in teenagers and people in their twenties, although it becomes more common in middle age. Usually it appears around the fifties, though very often there will have been warning aches and pains before then. Its incidence in the population gradually increases until 95 per cent of everyone over the age of 70 will suffer from it.

Not surprisingly, the joints most in use are the ones most likely to be affected, in particular those of the hands.

If you think about it, during your waking hours your fingers are in almost constant use — even in the most sedentary of jobs — and so osteoarthritis finds the finger joints, especially the terminal ones, a fertile field for attack. You may have noticed that many elderly people, almost always women, have swollen finger joints. The swellings, known as Herbenden's nodes, are soft at first, but later develop into bone.

The weight-bearing joints are also particularly prone to osteoarthritis, with the knees being the most susceptible. Hip replacement operations are now so common that it often seems as if it is the hip joint that suffers most from osteoarthritis. This is not so, it is just that the hip is better suited for surgical replacement than any of our other joints, not least the knee (see pages 58 and 61).

Little is known about the causes of osteoarthritis, but injury (generally referred to in medical circles as trauma) of the most trivial nature can sow the seeds of future trouble. For example, walking askew because of a limp can put unacceptable stress on a joint, which will eventually begin to degenerate and become arthritic.

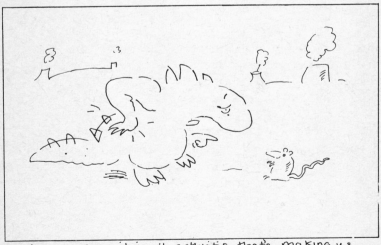

Are you sure it isn't arthritis that's making us extinct.

Having stated that, and made over-use and earlier traumas convenient scapegoats for causing osteoarthritis, disturbance of the body's chemicals can also bring on the disease. Ethnic factors, too, seem to have a bearing, as fewer people in tropical and sub-tropical countries suffer from osteoarthritis than in colder climates. It is impossible to say how far this is due to environmental factors, because little is really known about the cause of the disease.

Osteoarthritis is not confined to humans – it affects all vertebrates, animals without backbones. And it is not a disease of modern times, for traces of osteoarthritis have been found in the skeletons of Neanderthal men and, indeed, of dinosaurs!

Rheumatoid arthritis

Rheumatoid arthritis is a chronic disease, which can lead to gross deformity and ankylosis, or immobility of the joints. This is because the synovial membrane becomes thickened and may invade the joint, which makes it becomes swollen and extremely painful to move.

Unlike osteoarthritis, which is usually confined to a single joint, rheumatoid arthritis will attack several joints at the same time. It is very widespread, with

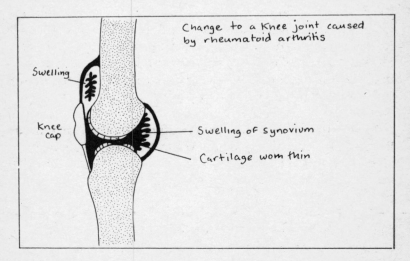

Change to a knee joint caused by rheumatoid arthritis

Swelling

Knee cap

Swelling of synovium

Cartilage worn thin

between 1 and 1½ million people in Britain suffering from it. For every two men with rheumatoid arthritis, there are four to five women. It usually appears during the first half of adult life, with the average age of onset being around 42. Seventy per cent of sufferers today are between 25 and 65 years of age. Rheumatoid arthritis, unlike osteoarthritis can, however, also attack children. In this form is it known as Still's Disease (see page 20).

In most cases, fortunately, the disease runs a comparatively mild course, but it can be so severe that the sufferer becomes badly disabled and even bed-ridden. Rheumatoid arthritis generally starts in the hands and feet before spreading to other joints. It does not follow a smooth, predictable course and the sufferer will have welcome periods of respite from pain when recovery will seem possible. Sadly these periods do not last long and the disease will always reassert itself.

Rheumatoid arthritis is usually far more complicated and difficult to control than osteoarthritis, because it is not, like that disease, sheerly a matter of wear and tear. But whichever you have, the effect will be similar – very considerable pain.

Gout
Gout is a disorder of the metabolism, the process whereby food is broken down into simple, digestible substances. It is caused when a person has too much uric acid in the blood, or when there is excessive secretion of uric acid in the kidney tubes. Both cause crystals of sodium biurate to be deposited in the affected joint, leading to intense pain.

Nine out of ten of those who suffer from gout are men. Women, for reasons unknown, have lower levels of uric acid in their blood; it is rare for women to get gout and then it is seldom likely to develop before the menopause.

Gout usually attacks a specific joint, most frequently the big toe, followed by the thumb. The condition is often associated with drinking too much alcohol or eating over-rich food. As a result, in Queen Victoria's day, the disease was depicted by cartoonists as most frequently affecting apoplectic colonels who, with a foot swathed in bandages and resting on a stool, brandished their malacca canes at cowering servants. Indeed, gout is still treated as a source of mirth by those who don't suffer from it. But, as you will know all too well if you have gout, there is nothing remotely amusing about it, for it can be extremely painful and the slightest movement, even an instinctive twitch at the slamming of a door, can cause piercing pain.

However, although the pain may be intense, you have

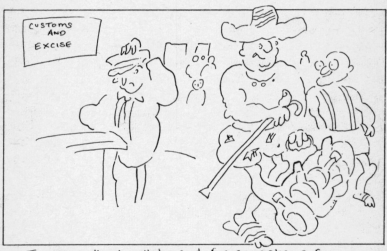

The gouty thumb will be good for smuggling a few miniature bottles next year.

the reassuring knowledge that the attack is unlikely to last more than a few days, as long as you take your pills (see page 43) and that is could be weeks, months, or even years before you have another attack.

Ankylosing spondylitis
Ankylosing arthritis is similar in many respects to rheumatoid arthritis, but instead of attacking several joints in different parts of the body, it generally just

affects the spinal column, the pelvic girdle and the
breastbone. The joints and the ligaments become ossified,
hardening into bone. The first joint to be affected is
usually the sacro-iliac, the articulation between the
sacrum – the division of the backbone to part of the pelvis
– and the hipbone.

The onset of ankylosing spondylitis is likely to be in
the forties and fifties. Men will often suffer from
inflammation of the prostate gland at the same time.

Unlike rheumatoid arthritis, however, ankylosing
spondylitis is more common in men than women. Recent
research, however, suggests that the difference is not as
wide as was formerly thought. The reason for the
apparent difference is psychological. Women are far more
likely than men to accept pain as 'just one of those things'
which has to be borne without complaint. As a result
women don't go to the doctor for help as often as men
and so don't enter the statistics.

The main problem if you have ankylosing spodylitis
is one of mobility. The spine becomes rigid, strictly
limiting all normal movement. The normal spinal column
is rather like a series of cotton reels threaded together,
but when you develop ankylosing spondylitis it is as if
an iron ram-rod had been thrust throught the holes,
leaving you with what has been called poker-back.

Psoriatic arthritis

Psoriatic arthritis, like gout, affects one in a thousand
of the population of Britain. That may seem a slight risk
to most of us, but the condition is a very real hazard for
those with the skin disease, psoriasis, as one in ten of
such sufferers are likely to develop this form of
arthritis.

The condition results in inflammation of the joint
uniting the pelvis and the hip-bone, which in normal
circumstances does not articulate, and in the spine and
its peripheral joints. Like rheumatoid arthritis, psoriatic
arthritis can erode cartilage and bone, causing
progressive instability.

Sometimes psoriatic arthritis becomes apparent before the skin disease itself.

Infective arthritis
Many arthritic conditions can be caused by known specific organisms and for convenience they are lumped together in medical reference books as 'specific infective arthritis'. Some of these conditions are extremely rare and are most likely to occur in the elderly, those already debilitated, or people who have rheumatoid arthritis or an infection, such as pneumonia, elsewhere in their body.

The commonest forms of infective arthritis are: *acute septic arthritis, tubercular arthritis, viral arthritis, gonococcal arthritis* and *syphilitic arthritis.*

Acute septic arthritis Acute septic arthritis occurs when bacteria such as streptococci, staphylococci and pneumococci intrude directly into a joint or are carried to a joint by infection in the blood.

Tubercular arthritis In the days when bovine tuberculosis was rife in Europe, tubercular infection of the bones and joints was extremely common. Now that dairy herds are free of the disease it is far less common.

Usually only one joint is affected and this is most likely to be in the spine, hip, knee or elbow. The pain is generally slight in the morning, but grows progressively worse as the hours pass. Although the pain is not as intense as in other forms of arthritis, it is still an acutely uncomfortable condition, for the joint will become swollen and stiff.

The incidence of tuberculosis has been dramatically reduced in developed countries, so that tubercular arthritis is now rare in these parts of the world, but it still attacks thousands in Asia and Africa where the disease is endemic. The condition is most commonly found in children and young adults.

Viral arthritis Arthritis in several joints may be found during an attack of rubella (German measles), but usually without any serious effects. It is also occasionally found in association with childhood illnesses such as mumps and chickenpox. It can also occur with smallpox, glandular fever and infective hepatitis.

Gonococcal arthritis Gonococcal arthritis develops from gonococcal urethritis, inflammation of the urethra, the channel through which urine is discharged from the bladder. Today, the infection can be rapidly treated by chemotherapy, so only one to two per cent of patients with gonococcal urethritis will develop gonococcal arthritis.

The arthritis usually follows within one to three weeks of an attack of the sexually transmitted disease and may affect several joints at the same time. The joints most likely to be affected are the knee, wrist, elbow and upper jaw. If the arthritis is confined to one joint, then it will be one of the larger joints which is in continual use. In miners, for example, it is most likely to develop in an elbow or wrist.

Syphilitic arthritis It is rare for syphilis to invade the joints, but when it does, it is usually because the disease has spread from the bones or it is a consequence of syphilitic disease of the nervous system.

Syphilis can now be rapidly and simply treated, so syphilitic diseases of joints and bones are rare in developed countries. When syphilitic arthritis occurs today, it is far more likely to be congenital than acquired.

Haemophiliac arthritis

This hereditary disease, which affects men but is carried by women, may cause a form of arthritis through haemorrhages, bleeding, into a joint. The knee is the joint most often affected, followed by the elbow or hip. The smaller joints are rarely affected.

The bleeding can be triggered by a very minor injury or strain. One single haemorrhage may be absorbed by the body without too much discomfort or damage, but only too frequently the first haemorrhage will be followed

by others which will, over the years, cause serious damage
to the synovial membrane and the cartilage.

Neuropathic arthritis

Neuropathic arthritis is a disease of the nervous system
which causes severe damage to joints and muscles. The
joints most commonly affected are the knee, spine, foot,
ankle and shoulder, in that order. Usually only a single
joint suffers harm. The disease renders the joint
concerned insensitive, so that you not only feel no pain
but are unaware that you have a joint that is being
damaged. A joint may, therefore, suffer repeated injury
or have to bear a greater strain than it is capable of
withstanding.

The effect on the joint closely resembles that of
osteoarthritis, but the destruction of the bone is likely
to be more severe. The disease involves the connective
tissues at several different sites, which suffer from
chronic inflammation as the normal structure is
destroyed. This destruction begins with the disease
infiltrating the synovial area. The synovial membrane
and sheath thicken and the inner surface becomes rough
and uneven, ridged with fine strands, which can grow
and intrude into the joints like the tentacles of an octopus.
They can only too easily become trapped in the joints
causing acute pain and aggravating the rheumatic
arthritic symptoms.

Still's Disease

Still's Disease (or inflammatory polyarthritis) is a rare
form of rheumatoid arthritis that affects children under
the age of 16. There is one major difference between this
and the adult form of rheumatoid arthritis: the patient
usually recovers fully.

2.
WHAT CAUSES ARTHRITIS?

For such a large 'family' of diseases that affect so many people, remarkably little is really known about the causes of the various types of arthritis. Indeed, this is one of the most frustrating aspects of the disease, both for sufferers and the medical profession.

There are, however, a number of factors that, while they may not actually or automatically cause a particular type of arthritis, are generally found in those who suffer from it. The presence of these factors may, therefore, indicate a predisposition towards the disease.

HEREDITARY FACTORS

Most of us will develop signs of wear and tear as we get older. Aches and pains are all too often accepted as an unavoidable part of the ageing process, instead of being recognized for what they often are – specific diseases. Such acceptance is particularly unwise if there is a family history of osteoarthritis. As with so many other diseases, if we really wish to avoid osteoarthritis we should choose our parents more carefully!

If your father and grandfather both suffered from osteoarthritis it does not automatically follow that you, too, will contract the disease, but you should at least be on the look-out for the symptoms (see page 25). Women are, in fact, more at risk than men, as there is tendency for osteoarthritis to pass from mother to daughter down the generations. This suggests that if the disease is clearly not caused by an injury, it is due to genetic and/or hormonal influences. Indeed, where there is a strong incidence of osteoarthritis in several family members, the symptoms may develop even when the victim is in his or her early thirties, although this is fortunately rare. In the meantime, if there is osteoarthritis in your family, be sure to keep your weight down, eat wisely and take regular, non-violent exercise.

Rheumatoid arthritis does not share this apparently hereditary characteristic with osteoarthritis, and if you have a close relative with the disease there is no reason to expect that you will develop it too.

Gout, however, is hereditary, although with this form of arthritis it is men rather than women who are most likely to be affected.

Ankylosing spondylitis also affects men rather than women, although women do get it. Investigation usually reveals a family history of the disease and, more often than not, you will find that a close relation, either your father or uncle, has it.

As seems to be the case in all arthritic troubles, it is impossible to trace an overall pattern and to state categorically that if your parents have, or had, any form of the disease then you, too, are bound to get it in your turn. But, at the same time, if there is a family history of it, you should be on the look out for the symptoms, so you can take steps to manage the disease, whichever it is, at the earliest possible stages (see Chapter 4).

DIET

At the moment there is no clear proof that diet plays a part in causing most forms of arthritis – despite what the advocates of many special diets claim to the contrary.

Considerable research is being done into this aspect of the disease (see page 56), but as yet nothing conclusive has emerged.

Gout, however, is the exception that proves the rule. As already mentioned (see page 15), gout has traditionally been caricatured as a disease of the rich. This was largely true in days gone by, because it was only the rich who could afford the food and drink that are likely to precipitate gout. Now, with greater affluence and more equality of living standards, we can all afford the disease, in dietary if not in health terms.

Foods that are high in uric acid should be avoided wherever possible if you have a close relative with gout. Among such foods are: offal, fish roes, and oily fish such as sardines, sprats and anchovies. Go easy, too, on thick, heavy gravies and all meat extracts.

The drinks that you would be well advised to steer clear of include port, madeira, rich heavy red wines and the strong and heavy beers. Champagne, too, has been found to bring on attacks of gout, though you may well find that the occasional celebratory glass will not leave you in acute pain the following day – but only you can discover that.

REPETITIVE STRAIN INJURIES

Repetitive strain injuries (RSI) can easily lead to arthritis if left without treatment. If you take part in any regular physical activity that involves a degree of unnatural stress on the body, such as modern dance, jogging, tennis or golf, you should be very aware of the dangers that RSI may pose to your health. They probably won't affect you now, but they may well later and they almost certainly will if you do nothing about them.

If a particular joint is over-used then tendonitis, inflammation of the tendon's sheath, sets in, with very painful results. You will find that the pain from the joint restricts the amount you can move it. Your wrist, for example, will become less and less mobile, until you can only use it in a very restricted manner.

Because of the restriction, the lubricating fluid does not flow between the surfaces of the joint's bones, so they become dry and lacking in nourishment. After a while, the lining of the joint begins to degenerate, and it will then not be long before arthritis sets in.

There is absolutely no reason why you should develop arthritis as a result of RSI. The condition is entirely preventable, but you must get early treatment. Follow the treatment conscientiously, and do the exercises that will probably be prescribed at the same time, and you should have few worries for the future.

MALFUNCTION OF THE IMMUNE SYSTEM

Another factor that may have a bearing on the cause of rheumatoid arthritis is a malfunctioning of the body's immune system. Research has not firmly established this, but there is certainly evidence that, for example, a virus infection could set off the disease.

We all have antibodies, protein substances usually circulating round our bodies in the blood, that will neutralize any harmful antigens (substances producing antibodies) that may have entered our bodies. However, abnormal antibodies are found in the blood of most victims of rheumatoid arthritis. Maybe it is these abnormal antibodies that are responsible for the inflammation and the changes this causes.

3. THE SYMPTOMS OF ARTHRITIS

OSTEOARTHRITIS

The symptoms of osteoarthritis usually appear very gradually, but may be accelerated by any minor injury such as a strain. At first there may be a slight stiffness, which you will probably ignore until it begins to interfere with particular movements, though even then it may only be noticeable after exercise. The degeneration of the joint is generally slow and you may not realize what is happening for months or indeed years. Many's the sufferer who has put up with considerable stiffness and pain before seeking medical advice on the basis of: 'I don't like to trouble you, doctor, it's only a few aches and pains . . .'

Doctors generally suspect osteoarthritis if their middle-aged or elderly patients complain of stiffness or where there is a deformity or signs of inflammation in a joint. Although osteoarthritis commonly affects a single joint, it can affect its symmetrical counterpart too, the other hip, for instance. Remember, too, that it's the weight-bearing joints that are most frequently affected.

You will probably not feel pain in the really early stages of the disease, provided that movement of the affected joint is strictly limited. It will, however, certainly make its presence felt the moment you try to force the joint beyond its usual range of movement. You will also find that pain tends to be worse after inactivity, for example after a night's rest, when getting out of bed may become a painful travail indeed. Sitting for hours almost motionless at a desk or in front of a television set is also likely to cause severe pain the moment you try to get out of the chair.

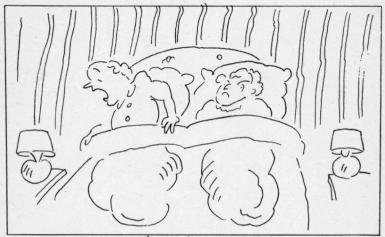

Arthritis my foot! You've had difficulty getting up for the last fifty years!

The affected joint gradually stiffens and the pain increases during movement until finally a stage may be reached when no useful movement of the limb is possible because of the extreme pain every time you attempt to move it. However, the course of the disease is rarely as severe as that, and usually it stops spontaneously before the disability becomes crippling.

Pain is really the important factor in osteoarthritis. Stiffness and deformity may irritate and frustrate, but pain is another matter. Not only can it destroy the ability to move, but it can also play on the mind until the sufferer can think of nothing else but the anguish to be endured.

Interestingly, the severity of the pain does not increase in proportion to the extent of the damage to the joint. Although X-rays can measure the amount of the damage, they can give little indication of the pain the patient is suffering. None of us feels pain in exactly the same way; pain is an individual experience. How we withstand it depends not only on our mood at that particular moment but also on environmental circumstances. If we are under pressure and highly emotional, it becomes far more difficult to put up with pain. When things are going well (apart, of course, from the fact of having osteoarthritis!) and we are living in comfortable surroundings, pain is far easier to bear.

Indeed the early stages of the disease may be far more painful than when the joint itself has deteriorated. As the cartilage begins to break down you may have severe pain, but later, when the cartilage has become eburnated, converted into a hard ivory-like substance, you are unlikely to have much pain.

RHEUMATOID ARTHRITIS

The one thing you can say with certainty about rheumatoid arthritis is that it is an entirely unpredictable disease. Usually it starts slowly and insidiously and is well-established before you realize what is happening to you. On the other hand it is not uncommon for the onset to be sudden, swift and obvious. In general, the smaller joints are attacked first, particularly the fingers. Then the disease will progress to the knees, elbows, ankles, shoulders and hips. However, it is not unusual for the large joints to suffer first, while the smaller ones escape until later in the disease's progress.

When rheumatoid arthritis attacks slowly, the first symptoms you are likely to notice will be slight pain, stiffness and tenderness around the affected joint. As in osteoarthritis, the pain and the stiffness will be most severe when you wake in the morning. The length of time the stiffness takes to wear off each day is a good pointer to the progress of the disease. Rheumatoid arthritis is tidal, ebbing and flowing. There may, indeed, be periods when you are totally free from pain.

In the beginning you may lose your appetite and with it some weight. You may also becomes anaemic, either because you have insufficient red blood cells or because the cells are deficient in haemoglobin. The first signs of anaemia are pallor of the skin and mucous membranes, especially in your lips and lower eyelids. You may feel weak and become giddy or faint; breathing may be difficult and you may also experience swollen ankles.

As the disease becomes established, the swelling will be more pronounced and the muscles will atrophy or waste, sometimes quite rapidly. Pain, stiffness and excruciating muscular spasms may hobble all movement. The skin will become taut, smooth and shiny. The hands and feet will sweat. The swollen joints will be red and hot with the skin apparently stretched tightly over them. There may also be an accumulation of 'water' around the swollen joint – this commonly occurs in the knee. The joints become spindly, especially those in the fingers. The swellings in the larger joints will seem disproportionately large because of the wasting of the muscle. Bending the joint becomes a problem because, without extreme care, dislocation can occur.

The deformities are easiest to see in the fingers because the joints have relatively little covering them. As the tissues around the joints are destroyed, so the joints will be difficult to control and keep in their normal positions, because the tendons that normally fulfil this function no longer have a stable joint on which to act. Indeed, the tendons themselves, under the tension of unstable joints, may rupture and so pull the joints into unnatural directions and awkward positions.

If you have rheumatoid arthritis you may develop a 'dropped finger'. Although the finger may be able to grip, it will remain closed after use and will not straighten voluntarily.

During the course of the disease, the cartilage of the

affected joint is transformed. First, instead of having a smooth, glossy appearance, the cartilage darkens to an unhealthy grey. Then, slowly it erodes, getting progressively thinner, until finally it disappears.

The inflammation, having attacked the membrane and the cartilage attached to the bone, then begins to affect the muscles. They will become severely wasted and may eventually be destroyed. This will result in loss of stability and control of movement, though sometimes this loss may be restored by surgical replacement of the damaged joint (see page 60).

As the muscles waste you may find nodules developing under your skin, particularly in your fingers and forearms. These are similar to nodules that have already formed in the muscles attacked by the disease. Interestingly, post-mortems carried out on patients with rheumatoid arthritis, even though it was not the cause of death, often reveal similar inflammatory nodules in the muscles of the heart.

GOUT

The base of the big toe is the most usual joint to be attacked by gout, perhaps because the blood flow there is more sluggish than in other joints.

Gout is usually acutely painful and the attacks sporadic. The start of an attack is often sudden and unexpected, although if you have had gout for some time you may learn to anticipate the onset of an attack. Sometimes it will be heralded by indigestion or discomfort in the bladder but, on the other hand, you may know an attack is in the offing because you feel unaccustomedly well – the peace before the storm.

Gout is a subtle enemy, often creeping up on you during the night and shocking you awake with the sheer ferocity of the pain. This pain increases in intensity until any movement – even movement by other people close to you in the room – will be almost beyond belief. It feels as if thumb-screws are being tightened around the joint and that if there is no relief the joint will burst through the skin. The joint swells and becomes red and angry, until putting on even a soft slipper is impossible.

You may find that gout is less painful during the day than at night – though this may be due more to the fact that there are more distractions during the day than any distinct medical cause. As an attack fades, so the swelling will go down and the colour of the skin return to normal, although it will peel and itch for a while.

An attack may last anything from a couple of days to a fortnight. The intervals between attacks may vary from weeks to years, but if the gout remains untreated the attacks will become more severe and more frequent.

When gout affects the hands instead of the toes, it follows a similar pattern. As well as the hands it may also attack the elbows and knees, sometimes triggering the onset of chronic arthritis.

ANKYLOSING SPONDYLITIS

In the early stages you will feel generally run-down and out of sorts and will lose weight. As movement in your spine becomes increasingly restricted, you will probably experience low back pain. As the disease increases in severity, so movement of the spine decreases until it sets and is rigid, from which the disease gets its nickname – poker-back. Because chest expansion is restricted, your breathing will be laboured and you will pant after even a slight exertion.

As the disease progresses so the low back pain will get worse and movement even more difficult. At this stage the vertebrae fuse into one stiff, bony column – a condition known as bamboo spine.

PSORIATIC ARTHRITIS

The first signs of the disease may be a slight pitting in your nails. The finger joints may swell and will feel hot and tender, or even painful, when you touch them.

ACUTE SEPTIC ARTHRITIS

Usually only one joint is affected, but this will become badly inflamed, making it swell and become painful. Pus may surround the joint and you will feel extremely ill, and will probably suffer from a high fever interspersed with violent cold shivering.

TUBERCULAR ARTHRITIS

Initially you will have relatively little pain, and then usually only in one joint – the knee is particularly common among adults, but elbows and hips are also at risk. As the disease progresses the pain will become worse, the joint stiffens and swells and is increasingly uncomfortable. The infection may spread into the surrounding muscles and tissues, where it will form abcesses. However, these are not like normal abcesses which are hot to the touch, but are known as cold abcesses. Apart from these there may be little outward sign of inflammation, but if treatment is delayed the destruction of the joint can be severe.

GONOCOCCAL ARTHRITIS

You will feel rotten and run a high fever two or three weeks after the symptoms of gonorrhoea have become apparent. Several of your joints are likely to be affected, usually the knee, wrist, elbow and upper jaw. However, if through your work or leisure activities you use one of your larger joints a great deal, it will be this one that is most at risk from this form of arthritis. The affected joints will be hot and tender to the touch, pus will form and you will be in quite severe pain.

SYPHILITIC ARTHRITIS

You will have a fever and feel generally low and out of sorts, and your joints will swell and be uncomfortable.

HAEMOPHILIAC ARTHRITIS

The haemorrhaging into a joint – usually the knee – causes pain and swelling. Normally the pain will not be too intense.

NEUROPATHIC ARTHRITIS

This form of arthritis will destroy a joint quite painlessly! The affected joint may becomes grossly swollen and can be manipulated into totally abnormal positions without you feeling any pain. So, start getting suspicious if you can suddenly do the lotus position when before you could hardly touch your toes!

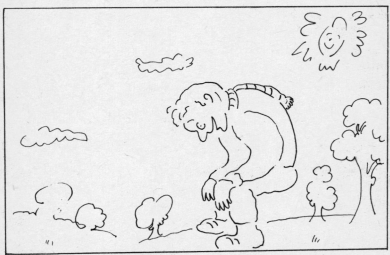

well I never thought I'd ever be able to touch my toes again.

STILL'S DISEASE

Still's Disease can appear at a very early age and may affect one or several joints. Fortunately it is usually quite easy to spot that there is something wrong with a child's movements even when it is still at the crawling stage.

4.
TREATMENT

As you will have gathered, not only are there a number
of different types of arthritis, but many of them do not
follow a predictable course. This, naturally, has a
profound effect on treatment. Together, you and your
doctor will have to work out a treatment regime that is
suitable for you. But, because there is such variety, both
within the various types of arthritis and in the individual
patient's response to treatment, there must be an element
of trial and error in the early stages of the treatment of
your condition. It is very important to remember this,
because low spirits and general despondency are two of
arthritis' more unpleasant side-effects. So if the first
treatment doesn't seem to be effective don't despair. It
is a pity and a further aggravation, but there are many
other types of drug, for example, at least one of which
will be of benefit to you.

Most treatment regimes are based on a combination
of drugs and exercise. The drugs are to control and reduce
pain, while exercise, properly prescribed of course,
maintains a degree of mobility and prevents joints seizing
up. But because of the trial and error necessarily involved,
it is very important that you tell your doctor if a drug
causes an unpleasant side-effect or that you've had to

stop doing the prescribed exercises because they caused even more pain and just made matters worse. However effective a drug or a set of exercises generally are, if they don't work for *you* they are no good! But, before you dismiss the usefulness of a particular drug to your condition, do make sure you are using it correctly. Follow the dosage instructions carefully and take care that you heed your doctor's warnings about any foods that you should avoid. Together, certain foods and drugs can be toxic.

There is, however, something that you can do for yourself which will certainly be of help – if you are overweight, do everything possible to lose those extra pounds. It won't cure your arthritis, but it will reduce the strain on joints that are under considerable stress already. Before you set about losing those unwanted pounds though, ask your doctor about the best way for you to do it – your body is having a hard time as it is, so you don't want to increase the pressure it is under by going on some ill-advised and badly thought out diet.

You may have heard, or even been told, that damp is bad for people who suffer from any type of arthritis. Indeed, traditional medicine always suggested that arthritis sufferers should eschew damp climates and recommended that winters, at least, should be spent where it was warmer – advice that was of little use to anyone who was not wealthy! There are, however, specialist rheumatologists who maintain that the climate, even when you are living in a semi-permanent mist, has not the remotest effect on any form of arthritis!

The situation is probably much more subtle. Cold and damp certainly depress the spirits and so reduce our ability to put up with pain. Sun can charm away blue devils and with the resurgence of our spirits, our aches and pains seem far less dreadful.

Most sufferers from arthritis, in whatever form, agree that the pain is likely to be most acute during the night, especially during those gaunt early morning hours when even the smallest, niggling problems are magnified into Goliath-sized insolubles. The discomforts of the day are aggravated by low spirits, bad body positions, uncontrolled movements during sleep, redistribution of body fluids and different hormone levels. And, of course, there are far fewer diversions during the night to take your mind off these worries, pains and discomforts.

Your doctor will prescribe drugs to help you sleep well at night without aggravating your arthritic condition. Drugs can help in these circumstances because they can reduce normal sleep movements. They do, however, have their disadvantages. Lack of movement can mean that you wake up with stiff joints. A combination of sedatives and anti-inflammatory drugs will help control this problem. Night cramps, too, can be excruciating, but can be dealt with effectively by drugs.

Then, apart from those low spirits during the early hours, there is the problem of general depression. Pain during the day is bad enough, but add to this exhaustion through lack of sleep, perhaps social problems caused by the disease (problems of mobility, for example), and the frustration of having to concentrate all your physical and mental powers to make even modest movements – movements you previously took for granted – and the outcome will very likely be depression. When you reach this pitch there are anti-depressant drugs to help you. And, nearer to home, if your friends and family tell you to 'Snap out of it', do try to explain to them that you can't do so without help, and that their attitude is *not* the help you mean!

Because so many people suffer from the different forms of arthritis, a great deal of research is going on into causes and treatments. As a result, a new drug or some other 'breakthrough' in treatment is often given extensive coverage in the media. This is a pity because it raises the hopes of many sufferers, who ask their doctor for the new drug only to be told that it is not suitable for them or their form of arthritis. It is difficult, but try not to let yourself fall into this trap.

OSTEOARTHRITIS

In the early stages your doctor will probably prescribe non-steroid anti-inflammatory drugs (NSAI) to reduce the inflammation of the affected joints. And you can use electric blankets and/or pads to apply heat generally or locally, as heat is always comforting and relaxing. These appliances should be examined and, where necessary, serviced at least once a year.

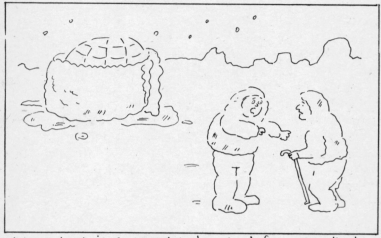

I Know heat is supposed to be good for our arthritis, but was that a good place to put the electric blanket?

Physiotherapy will also play an important role in your treatment, as it both strengthens the muscles and provides stability for the joints. Exercise should, however, be avoided when joints are swollen or inflamed. Indeed, when the condition is severe, the best treatment is rest in bed with aspirin to relieve the pain.

It is also important to get advice about ways in which you can adapt your home to prevent causing unnecessary stress and discomfort. Your bed is, of course, quite crucial in this respect (see page 86). Such adaptations have the extremely important benefit of helping you maintain a degree of independence. And there are few things more damaging to morale than finding you are no longer able to lead an independent existence.

In the advanced stages of osteoarthritis your doctor will prescribe drugs to reduce the pain but, sadly, that is all they can do. They cannot replace or rebuild damaged or worn out joints. Injecting corticosteroids into the osteoarthritic joints sometimes works effectively on the inflammation, and your doctor may suggest this. However, even if it is effective, this is not a long-term treatment as too many injections can themselves damage the joints. Aspiration of the swollen joints to let out the excess fluid will relieve the pressure and pain. But aspiration, despite the usual reassurances that 'this won't hurt for more than a moment . . .', is not a pleasant experience, and it, too, is not a long-term solution.

When all treatments have failed, and the pain is making life insupportable, remember that there are replacement operations. They are major operations and no surgeon will undertake them lightly, but they are becoming increasingly common (especially hip and knee replacements, see pages 59 and 61) and the success rate is encouragingly high.

RHEUMATOID ARTHRITIS

There is no sure cure for rheumatoid arthritis, so treatment inevitably has to be regular and prolonged. Indeed, you may well find that your doctor refers to the 'management' rather than the 'treatment' of your disease.

The commonest drug used in treating rheumatoid arthritis is calcium aspirin – soluble aspirin. Generally this is the first line of defence because it effectively kills pain and reduces inflammation. The calcium added to aspirin counteracts what otherwise might be a gastric irritant leading to nausea or even, eventually, to ulceration. But the combination still causes some side-effects: gastric pain, tinnitus (ringing in the ears) or the vomiting of blood may occur if the course is carried on for too long. But as these side-effects are well-known, your doctor will be on the lookout for them and will be unlikely to prescribe aspirin long enough for them to affect you.

When rheumatoid arthritis is really acute, your joints will become swollen and still, you will feel extremely unwell and have a temperature. At this stage rest is essential, be it in hospital or at home. As with osteoarthritis, take great care over the type of bed you have. If you have not already done so, and if it is possible, do try to get an appropriate bed (see page 86). Bedclothes, which normally merely provide warmth, can become an intolerable weight, especially when the knee joints are affected. Use a cradle to support the bedclothes and prevent them pressing on your painful joints.

Never put a pillow under your knees to reduce pain and discomfort. It will probably do this quite effectively, but it can also cause flexing deformities. You should keep your legs as straight as possible, but also allow them to be mobile — stillness can lead to thrombosis (formation of blood clots which may eventually cause heart problems).

Nevertheless, certain risks must be accepted during some stages of the disease. And during the most painful times it may be necessary to immobilize the joint using light splints or plaster of Paris, but only, of course, under medical supervision (see page 54).

If you do have to spend time in bed, don't fret and rail against your fate, put the time to good use instead. For a start you can get to know your physiotherapist and plan just how you are going to work together in the coming months. As well as keeping the muscles controlling the joints mobile and maintaining joint movement, you will have a good opportunity to find out about and understand the management of your disease and its treatment. The success or failure of the treatment may well depend on your co-operation, because in this, as in many other diseases, treatment is not something that is done to a passive you — you have to participate as actively as you can (always, of course, following the advice of your doctor and physiotherapist).

No exercise regime should be introduced without a full explanation of the basic principles behind the plan and, most important, what the side-effects are likely to be. If you don't understand, ask. After all, it is your body and you are the one who is suffering.

Invariably the disease regresses and as the pain and discomfort lessen, then the affected joints need not be cosseted quite so much. They may be exercised once it has been established that movement does not revive the pain. At this stage of treatment you will probably be encouraged to get up and out of bed for increasingly long periods. You may be nervous about this at first, fearing a recurrence of the pain that caused you to be in bed in the first place. You won't be the first (or, sadly, the last) sufferer from rheumatoid arthritis to feel like this, but try to overcome the fear and follow the encouraging advice, because spending too long in bed, when it is no longer necessary, will just increase the likelihood of stiff, immobile joints and heart problems.

At some time in the course of the disease your doctor may suggest a course of drugs to control the pain and inflammation. As in osteoarthritis, you may be prescribed corticosteroids. These are injected directly into affected joints and, again, though often effective, this is not a long-term treatment.

Injections of gold salts may also be effective, but there must be gaps of several months between courses as they sometimes cause toxic reactions, resulting in skin rashes, a low white blood cell count, mouth ulcers and even kidney disease.

D-penicillin, which has great similarity with gold salts, has been introduced over the last ten years as an accepted treatment. One of its advantages over gold salts is that it can be taken orally. As with other drugs, be alert and on the watch for the first signs of any side-effects, which include skin rashes. If such warnings are ignored the drug can cause kidney damage and abnormal blood conditions, leading to wasting.

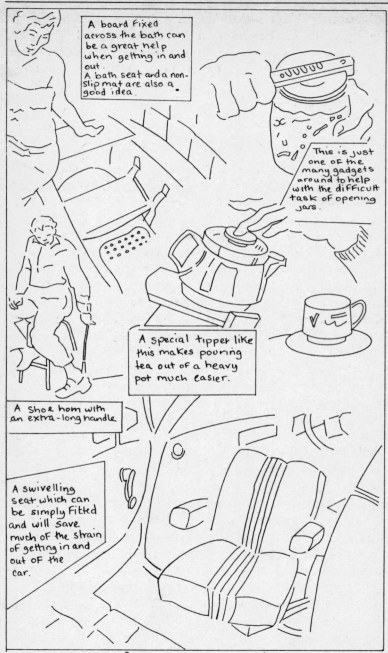

Several ways of coping with arthritis.

Drugs developed to treat malaria have also been used successfully and can lead to remissions lasting for as long as three months at a time. However, these drugs can cause eye trouble and if you are on such drugs you must have regular examinations of your eyes by a trained opthalmologist.

GOUT

Gout can now be treated most effectively, and provided you follow your doctor's instructions you should be able to prevent the worst of the disease's misery, if not avoid it altogether.

Gout is a disease with a long history – the ancient Greeks suffered from it. They also discovered what, until recently, was the only drug that proved effective in treatment: colchicine, which is derived from the meadow saffron or autumn crocus. Today, however, colchicine is still used, but is just one of several drugs used in treating the disease. As before, be alert for any side-effects from the drugs you have been prescribed. (One drawback of colchicine is that it can cause severe diarrhoea.)

Once it is obvious that you have a predisposition to gout – in other words you have had an attack of it! – there are a number of things you can do to make another attack less likely. The first is, if possible, lose weight – but ask your doctor's advice first about a suitable diet for you. Secondly, avoid the types of food high in uric acid mentioned on page 23. Thirdly, if you know you have high levels of uric acid in your blood (and your doctor will probably have given you a blood test to establish this soon after your first attack of gout) avoid having blow-outs of food and/or drink. Small meals regularly is sound advice for anyone, but is really essential for the gout sufferer. Finally, and probably most effective of all, is treatment to reduce the level of uric acid in your blood. This, of course, is a long-term treatment and can only be prescribed by your doctor. But, once prescribed, it is up to you to be conscientious and follow the instructions

– which may well include not taking these drugs during an attack of gout (should you suffer another one.)

ANKYLOSING SPONDYLITIS

The disease itself will not be treated, but the pain and swelling can be controlled by drugs in the same way as they are for rheumatoid arthritis. You will also have physiotherapy to help you improve your posture and make the most of what movement is still available to you. If one or both of your hips are involved, surgery may be necessary (see page 58).

It is absolutely essential that you have a firm, non-sagging mattress.

PSORIATIC ARTHRITIS

The symptoms will be treated with anti-inflammatory drugs, while the 'parent' disease, the psoriasis, is being treated.

ACUTE SEPTIC ARTHRITIS

First you will be treated with a course of antibiotics. If, however, these are not very effective, it may be necessary to drain the fluid from the affected joint every day. This technique, known as aspiration, uses a needle inserted in the joint to drain off the fluid. During this procedure, antibiotics may be injected directly into the joint.

TUBERCULAR ARTHRITIS

Treatment with antitubercular drugs is the usual procedure. Very occasionally, the affected joint will be fused surgically to render it rigid. This process, called arthrodesis, is, as you can imagine, very much a last resort used only when the progress of the disease has caused severe damage to the joint.

GONOCOCCAL ARTHRITIS

The treatment is with penicillin.

SYPHILITIC ARTHRITIS

Penicillin is the treatment for this disease, too.

HAEMOPHILIAC ARTHRITIS

The treatment is the same as that for the 'parent' disease, haemophilia, in other words blood transfusions when necessary. The affected limb(s) will also be rested and supported with the aid of splints and firm bandaging.

This treatment will be followed by a routine of gentle exercising to reduce the likelihood of subsequent disability.

NEUROPATHIC ARTHRITIS

The treatment will be very similar to that of the treatment for the symptoms of osteoarthritis.

STILL'S DISEASE

This disease is quite likely to disappear gradually without any medical intervention. Nevertheless it is important that the symptoms are treated. The affected joint(s) must be protected by splints, while gentle exercises are maintained to avoid later damage. You should give your child every comfort and understanding, but it is also very important to encourage him or her to be as active as possible, so that he or she will be able to lead a physically active life.

PHYSIOTHERAPY

After arthritis has been diagnosed and drugs prescribed, the physiotherapist may well become more important in your life than either your doctor or consultant. During the weeks in hospital or at home and confined to bed or a chair, the physiotherapist will probably be your most regular visitor. And, unlike hard-pressed doctors, physiotherapists will make time to listen to your woes and to explain the whys and wherefores of the exercises you have been advised to do. A good physiotherapist will regard answering your questions as being quite as important as monitoring your physical progress.

The aim of physiotherapy is to maintain and improve the range of movements in your joints, this the therapist does by working on those muscles that control the joints, as well as providing them with the vital stability without which we'd be totally unco-ordinated. As well as telling you and explaining to you what you must do for yourself to retain as much movement as you can, the physiotherapist will take over – either with massage or with electrical apparatus – when you are unable to do exercises yourself.

The exercises used in physiotherapy are many and various. Those described below are just a few of the many, so don't worry if your physiotherapist doesn't prescribe any of them for you – and don't try any of them without first asking the advice of your doctor or your physiotherapist. And *never* do any exercise, even if it has been prescribed for you, if it increases pain in the joint it is supposed to be helping.

Exercises for hands

You should exercise arthritic hands separately so that you concentrate on each in turn. Otherwise, subconsciously, you will allow your best, strongest hand, to assert itself over the weaker, and so be exercising the hand which needs it least.

All the hand exercises are comparatively simple. One of the easiest, yet most effective, is merely to clench the fist as tight as possible and then open it to its fullest extent with the fingers spread wide. Then relax it. Repeat with the other hand. And so on. The great advantage of this exercise is that you can do it any time and anywhere without attracting attention.

Wrist exercises

There are very few exercises for strengthening your wrists and increasing their mobility. These two very simple ones are probably as good as any. In the first one, sit down and keep your elbows close to your sides. Then bend each wrist in turn as far back as possible before straightening it again and relaxing. In the second one,

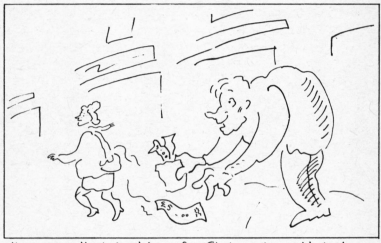

Its an excellent condition for finding the odd lost five pound note. It gives me a chance to do my hand exercises as well.

sit as before and then rotate each wrist in turn in as near a circular movement as possible.

Elbow exercise

The elbow is a hinge joint, and so is best exercised by a simple up and down movement. Again, exercise each elbow separately so that you can concentrate on each one individually. Sit as comfortably as possible on a chair (an upright one is best) with your feet flat on the floor, and your upper arms close to your sides. Clench one of your fists, bend your elbow and raise the lower part of your arm until it as close to your chin as possible. Lower your forearm, relax, and repeat several times before exercising the other elbow.

Shoulder exercises

Cultivate the Gallic shrug – that is certainly the simplest, and probably the best, exercise you can give your shoulders! Shrug them (both together this time) as high as you can, lower them, relax and repeat.

Another good exercise for the shoulders is to draw them as far back as possible, so that the shoulder-blades are almost touching. Relax and then repeat the movement.

Neck exercises

There are several effective exercises you can do to help strengthen and maintain mobility in your neck. They also have the advantage of being very easy.

For the first exercise sit straight upright with your face forward. Then keeping your head and neck erect, turn your face slowly but firmly to the right, so that your eyes are focussed over your right shoulder. Pause a moment, then turn back to the front. Relax. Repeat the exercise to the left. Relax, repeat, and so on.

Remain sitting upright for the second exercise, with your head erect and facing forward. Nod, bringing your chin down close to your chest. Straighten your neck to the upright position. Relax. Next move your head backwards as far as possible until your eyes are looking up to the ceiling. Straighten. Relax. Then repeat the sequence.

For the third exercise sit upright, but drop your chin onto your chest. Begin to rotate your head slowly so that it 'rolls' round in a complete circle. Keep this up until you have managed to do several circuits. Pause and relax. Drop your chin again and roll your head in the other direction. Pause and relax. Repeat several times in each direction.

When you first do this exercise it may seem, and even sound, as though there are several drummers playing on your upper vertebrae. Don't worry! But equally don't overdo the exercise. The more frequently, and regularly, you do the exercise the less discomfort there will be. Most people, even those in their early forties, will find that head rotation is uncomfortable at first.

Neck exercises, particularly of a rotary nature, can sometimes have bad results for arthritic patients, having disturbing effects on balance. They can cause giddiness and nausea. At the first sign of such effects, the exercises should be discontinued.

Feet exercises
Lie flat on your bed with your feet together and the toes pointing towards the ceiling. Curl the toes of your right foot as tightly as possible. Straighten them and relax. Now do the same with the other foot. Relax. Repeat with each foot in turn, relaxing between each exercise.

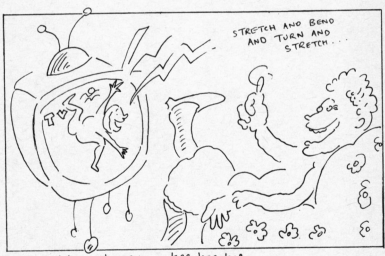

Stretch on honey ... hee hee hee.

Exercise for the ankles
Lie flat on your bed, again with your feet together and toes pointing to the ceiling. Extend your right foot until the toes are pointing down towards the end of the bed. Straighten your foot and relax. Repeat with the left foot.

Straighten and relax. Repeat with the right foot and so on.

Exercises for the knees

Lie flat on your bed with your toes towards the ceiling and your knees together. Bend your right leg up, until the sole of the foot is resting on the bed and the knee is fully flexed. Straighten the leg and relax. Repeat with the left leg.

Relax and then repeat the exercise with each leg in turn.

If you do not suffer too much from limitation of movement, try this rather more complicated exercise. Lie on your bed as before and draw up your right leg until it is fully flexed. Now, start to rotate both legs as if you were riding a bicycle, keeping the knees constantly on the move. Pause to relax after a few rotations and then repeat.

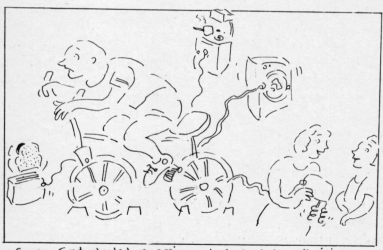

Since Fred started exercising to help his arthritis we've had no electricity bills at all.

Hip exercises

Lie flat on the bed with your toes to the ceiling. Bring both legs up until the knees are fully flexed and touching each other. Now spread your knees as widely as possible. Close. Relax. Repeat. This is not a particularly easy exercise at the best of times, so do not overdo it – but, at the same time, don't give up after the first attempt!

Exercises for the spine
Never do these exercises, or any other, for the spine unless you have first consulted your doctor or physiotherapist. For the first exercise stand with your hands straight down beside you. Smoothly and gently start to bend forward, sliding your hands down the sides of your legs as you bend. When you have bent as far forward as possible, pause a moment, and then just as slowly and smoothly start to straighten up. Straighten, relax and repeat.

Start the second exercise standing up straight with your hands on your hips. Slowly bend sideways as far to the right as possible without strain. Straighten up. Relax. Repeat the exercise bending to the left. Straighten, relax and repeat.

Again, stand upright with your hands on your hips. Bend forward and then begin to rotate your body from the waist – in the same way as the ankle is rotated in the ankle exercise above. After a few circuits relax. Straighten up and then repeat. If it is very difficult, start by doing one or two very slow gentle circuits.

INTRA-SONIC PAIN RELIEF THERAPY

Research into the effects on the body of exposure to various forms of electro-magnetic wave emissions began in the 1930's. Professor Dr Erwin Schliephake in Germany became especially intrigued with the therapeutical possibilities of using audible sound frequencies. His experiments and research in this field are the basis of today's intra-sonic pain relief treatment.

A vibrating disc sends out waves. Those detectable by the human ear are termed intra-sound (below this range the waves are infra-sound and above ultra-sound). These waves provide an efficient form of deep massage which stimulates the tissues and spurs the blood circulation to the treated area. In effect this means giving nature a helping hand.

Intra-sound pain relief therapy promotes the healing process. It can be directed onto the exact spot needed by altering the speed or changing the sound-head. The sound-head is the osculating disc which you place on the desired area. You do not have to press it hard but merely make contact with the skin. It can be flat or thimble-shaped to reduce the area of contact.

Intra-sonic pain relief can be used to treat many ailments such as arthritis, low back pain, sprains and fractures. It also affords relief to many suffering from migraine. From my personal experience it can work wonders for arthritic fingers and hands. It had been thoroughly tested by medical authorities and is perfectly safe and has no side effects.

The only word of warning necessary is that this treatment should *not* be used by anyone with a pacemaker or in cases where the patient is suffering from pain of unknown origin in the lower legs. In the latter instance, medical advice should, of course, be sought.

HYDROTHERAPY

Hydrotherapy enables you to carry out exercises that would be quite impossible on dry land because a limb, supported by water, becomes almost weightless. As well as helping you to exercise fully in a way nothing else can, hydrotherapy is a wonderful post-operative muscle strengthener.

Ideally, exercises are carried out in a large, shallow, warm, swimming pool, constructed so that patients can walk down to the depth they require, although a hoist and chair can be used if walking isn't yet possible for you. Underwater, a painful joint may be exercised with far less effort and far less pain than at home.

There are, of course, many methods of nursing a joint

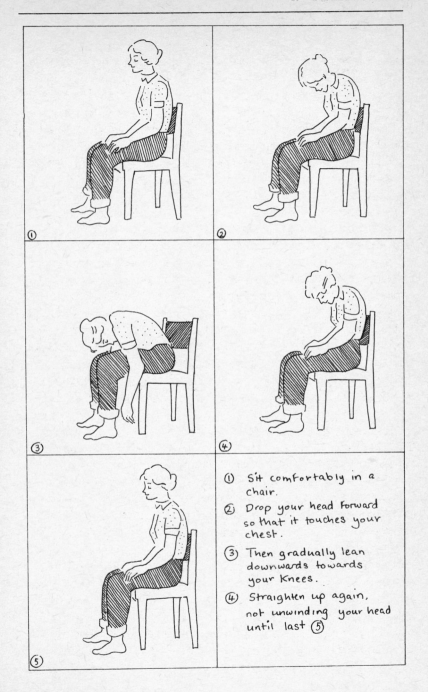

① Sit comfortably in a chair.

② Drop your head forward so that it touches your chest.

③ Then gradually lean downwards towards your knees.

④ Straighten up again, not unwinding your head until last ⑤

and teaching it to start working again, but hydrotherapy must be the most pleasant. But therein lies a danger. The feeling of comfort and relaxation can be so strong that unless the physiotherapist acts as a sergeant-major you may be tempted to do too much. It is also important that, however fit you may feel after hydrotherapy, you should take a rest, preferably swathed in warm towels and lying on a comfortable bed.

Except in the early stages of rheumatoid arthritis, swimming is generally an excellent treatment for arthritis, so do use your local swimming-pool as often as possible. And try not to feel self-conscious if you are scarred by the surgeon's scapel or have been deformed by arthritis. Take comfort from someone who is both scarred and deformed – you'd be amazed just how unobservant and uninterested most people are.

APPARATUS

Splints and plaster of Paris are used when rheumatoid arthritis attacks become so severe that a limb must be immobilized.

Splints may also be used to provide support and so relief from pain in an inflamed joint, particularly wrists, knees and ankles. Splints are also used if a hand is severely affected.

Never ever use a splint or try to set a joint with plaster of Paris yourself. Both these forms of treatment tend to be regarded as rather desperate remedies when the disease is particularly bad and must, like any other treatment, be used only under close medical supervision.

HEAT TREATMENT

Heat treatment is sometimes called diathermy or electrotherapy and can be very helpful in relieving the pain suffered by most victims of the various types of arthritis.

Modern heat treatment is based on diathermy – the passage of a high frequency electric current through the skin and the tissues of the joints beneath. Heat is generated by the electrical resistance of the tissues to the current. If large electrodes are used to attach the wires to the skin the heat is diffused over a large area.

If smaller electrodes are used instead, the heat can be localized and so focussed onto a small area. (Thus it can also be used to cauterize. During operations today diathermy is used to seal bleeding points, so allowing surgeons a clear operating field. Before diathermy, every single bleeding point had to be tied, which involved many, many, clamps and the surgeon operating amongst a forest of metal.)

Some rheumatologists state unequivocally that heat does little except improve the spirits, but to set against this is the theory that the two sensations, pain and heat, compete for our attention. Sometimes heat wins, driving out pain for perhaps an half hour. Being free from pain for even such a short time is not to be lightly dismissed; for freedom from chronic pain, even if only for a few minutes, gives us the chance of regenerating our powers

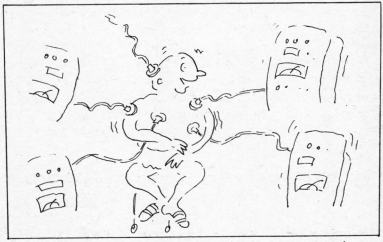

I'm glad this electro-therapy is on your electricity bill.

of resistance.

Heat treatment has another valuable use. If muscles have been out of use for a long period, the patient may have forgotten how to use them. Electrotherapy can take over and motivate the muscles when the patient's brain fails to do so. Tiny electrical shocks – not very unpleasant – can make the muscles contract. This helps exercise the muscles and reminds the patient how to use them. This is not a DIY treatment, but must be applied by a physiotherapist.

DIET

There are almost as many diets that are claimed to cure arthritis as there are different types of the disease. Each diet has its champions, and very vociferous they usually are!

These crusaders pressurize every arthritis sufferer they meet that they should adopt their own particular nostrum. But diet must be an individual choice and never be tempted to embark on a new diet without first seeking medical advice. Caution is vital at the best of times, but it is even more necessary when you are already unwell. Anything which affects your health must not be embraced until all its possible side-effects have been studied. It is little use dieting because you are too heavy if afterwards you are too weak to enjoy yourself. What is more, it is no use rushing enthusiastically into a new regime only to be disappointed.

But, despite this warning note, there is little doubt that arthritis may be affected by allergies to certain foods and research has indicated that some groups of food, particularly flour products, are more likely than others to be the culprits.

The difficulty for the individual is finding out which particular item is causing the trouble. It certainly isn't easy to identify one particular food merely by omitting a substance from your diet and waiting to see if you feel better. If you listed everything you ate in the course of a week, you'd probably find the list contained several hundred different items. Dropping one food for several days is not going to tell you much, and it is almost impossible to state categorically that any easing of pain is due to avoiding a certain food and not to some other cause: change of environment, raising of spirits through good news, improvement in the weather or the natural regression of the disease.

However it is possible, under carefully controlled medical supervision, to discover if an allergy to a particular food, or group of foods, is a cause of the arthritic condition. Sadly, the treatment is not widely available, but the principle behind it is as follows.

Before the investigation begins properly, the patient must be cleansed of the recent intake of food and this entails a very bland diet and fasting. Once this cleansing, detoxifying process is over, the patient starts on a specially monitored diet.

Certain groups of food are excluded, group by group. For instance one of the commonest groups found to conceal the cause of the problem is the flour products.

As each group of foods is withdrawn, the patient is asked to try and assess how he or she feels. There are three variables: pain by day, pain by night and morning stiffness. Pain is always difficult to assess accurately, and arthritis, with its remissions of pain, makes matters worse. As a result, if you do feel better the reason may have nothing at all to do with what you've been eating. Generally, when trying to record pain reaction to any treatment, a four-point scale is used to try and measure the pain over each 24-hour period. Records are kept of the number of joints affected. As well as recording the patient's subjective reactions, the doctor records his or her own findings when exerting pressure on the joint and noting the effect on the patient.

So one selected group of foods is withdrawn from the diet. Then if after a period there is no change for better or worse and the pattern of pain does not seem to have altered, that group of foods is believed to be innocent and restored to the diet and another group eliminated in its place. There are a limited number of groups of food and so, if diet is responsible, it will not be so very long before the guilty group is identified.

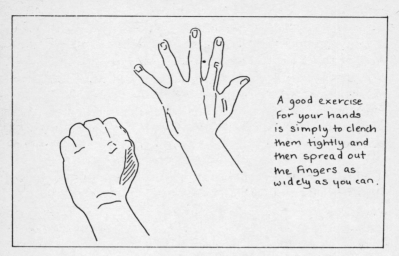

A good exercise for your hands is simply to clench them tightly and then spread out the fingers as widely as you can.

Once the group has been identified, individual foods from within that particular group are withdrawn. Eventually, by a process of elimination, the villain of the piece is finally exposed. It is a process which cannot be hurried. It takes time and needs methodical recording. Of course, there is no reason why you shouldn't carry out this form of research on your own, but clearly what has taken experts under scientifically controlled conditions months to achieve will take you far, far longer.

SURGERY

Surgery is, of course, the last resort and, despite the almost miraculous results of most replacement operations, should never be embarked upon until absolutely necessary. However sophisticated and efficient surgical techniques may have become and however cleverly designed the replacement joints, the removal of a human joint and its replacement with a man-made device is always major surgery.

The operation to replace arthritic hips has been considerably refined since it was first introduced in the 1930s, and its success rate is high. The prosthesis, the man-made replacement, is now really quite small – the first ones, logically enough, were the same size as the parts of the joint they were replacing. Originally, too, both parts – the ball on its spike and the cup-like socket into which it fitted – were made of steel. Today the Charnley Prosthesis, which is the one most commonly used, replicates the head of the femur (the ball of the thigh bone) in stainless steel, while high-density polyethylene replicates the acetabulum, the socket in the hip into which the head of the femur fits. This reduces friction and metal fatigue, which sometimes caused all-metal prostheses to loosen or breakdown altogether. A type of cement is used to fixed the prosthesis firmly into the bone of the hip, while the femoral ball is mounted on a metal spike which is driven into the shaft of the thigh bone (the femur) once the damaged part of the bone has been sawn off.

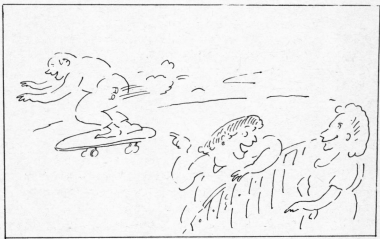

When he got his new hip replacement he asked for it to be turbo-charged.

You won't, of course, be aware of what is going on during the operation, but all too soon after you've come around from the general anaesthetic you'll become aware of the major problem that immediately follows hip operations: keeping your legs straight. Dislocation of your prosthesis is a danger and very real possibility in the days following a hip operation – any sudden movement can jerk the ball and the socket apart. So, for the first few nights after your operation, you will have to sleep on your back with a wedge-shaped pillow between your legs to prevent you crossing them. It is also vital in these early days that you don't cross one leg over the other – night or day.

This is not as simple as it sounds, because crossing one ankle and resting it upon the other has become almost a reflex action. The nurses on orthopaedic wards have to adopt sergeant-major tactics to remind patients of the risks!

The physiotherapist plays a major role in helping you avoid dislocation. You will be taught how to avoid incorrect movements in the early post-operative days, and given exercises to strengthen the muscles supporting and controlling the prosthesis, which you will have to continue after you have left hospital. The physiotherapist will also guide you as you take your first tentative steps and then, triumphant day, tackle the stairs. Indeed, you will not be discharged from hospital until you have overcome these two hurdles: walking and climbing stairs. So don't worry if you live on your own – you will be mobile, if slowly, when you are sent home. Even so, you are unlikely to be in hospital for more than two weeks, which in itself is a comforting reassurance of just how routine and successful this operation is.

The reasons surgeons concentrated from the start of replacement surgery on the hip are easy to understand. The hip is a comparatively straighforward ball and socket joint when studied from an engineering point of view. And the engineering aspect must not be overlooked because the engineer has played a major role in the development of replacement surgery; indeed, in the early days the engineer's ingenuity and imagination were every bit as important as the surgeon's skill. In fact, the engineer stood at the surgeon's elbow by the operating table to advise exactly where the prosthesis could be most effectively cemented into place.

Hip replacement proved so successful that it was only logical that surgeons should turn their attention to other joints.

The knee was the natural successor. However, the knee is not nearly as straightforward a joint as the hip for there is no surrounding socket to prevent a rotatory movement and so provide stability for the prosthesis. So as well as giving painless, smooth movement, the replacement must also provide a very firm, stable base. As in the hip operation, steel and plastic are used to reduce wear and tear. Recovery may take a little longer but is still extremely rapid when compared to most operations. It has taken some time to master the problems posed by this operation, but it is now carried out almost as routinely as the hip replacement operation.

The ankle is more complicated still, for although it, too, is a hinge joint so far as the up and down movement is concerned, it also has to rotate, as well as bear a considerable amount of weight. However research is continuing and knowledge increasing, and there was a time quite recently when no joint could be replaced.

Wrist replacement is very seldom undertaken or even considered, because to make it firm and steady much of its movement would have to be sacrificed. And there is little to be gained in operating on the wrist when, as is highly likely, the fingers are themselves gnarled with rheumatism and unable to grasp anything firmly.

The success of replacing finger joints depends largely on the extent of the deformity. The surgeon may operate on a hand and improve movement, but if the deformity is of long standing, there is little likelihood that it can be refashioned to its original state. If, however, the disease is confined to the knuckle joints, replacement can work wonders.

Some hospitals even carry out knuckle replacements – the prosthesis looks rather like a miniature sea urchin – in out-patients' departments under a local anaesthetic. If this is how yours are going to be treated don't worry; a screen is raised so you won't see what the surgeon is doing with the scalpel! After the sea urchins have been inserted and the wound sewn up, your hand will be bandaged and the arm supported in a sling. After a few days you will return to out-patients' to have the stitches removed, and leave with an almost new hand. But certainly at first, don't demand too much of those new joints.

The elbow joint, like the ankle, has not only to provide an up and down movement but must also be able to rotate. To date the replacement of elbow joints has been more a saga of failure than a history of success. It is a major joint which has to sustain continual and heavy strain. After all, each of your arms weighs over a pound and a half before you start lifting heavy objects. So, for the time-being at least, surgical replacement of the elbow joint is not recommended.

Shoulder movement can be improved by surgery, but the replacement of the whole joint would, at the present time, pose far too many problems. However, a prosthesis not unlike that for the hip has been devised in which a man-made ball and socket joint is set into the humerus (upper arm bone) and scapula (shoulder blade) respectively. As you will know, if you have arthritis affecting this part of the body – even this limited replacement could be better than none at all.

The importance of the engineering aspect of joint replacement must not be forgotten, for it does not end with the design and manufacture of the replacement joint. Wear and tear must always be considered and the man-made replacements must be fully tested, before being put into use, to see how they will react to constant movement. This means devising machines to emulate the movements of the joints which are to be replaced. Watch your own

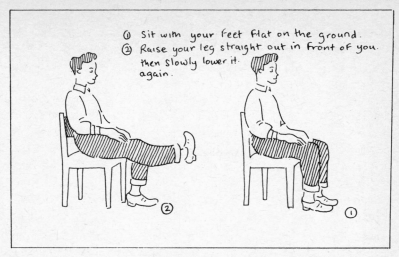

① Sit with your feet flat on the ground.
② Raise your leg straight out in front of you. then slowly lower it again.

fingers for a short time and you'll be amazed to realize they are in almost continual use, seldom are they still for more than a second at a time. It is indeed a tribute to Nature's engineering that, unless we have arthritis, they usually last our life time. Human engineers have to test and retest their inventions lest patients have to undergo repeat operations.

Post-operative infection is no longer the danger it used to be. Thanks to antibiotics and improved surgical techniques there is very little to fear from this aspect of surgery.

That other enemy, thrombosis, has also lost much of its power with the introduction of modern post-operative nursing. The nurses really aren't being callous when they make you get out of bed when it seems as if you've only been out of the operating theatre a few minutes! Shock, too, has been minimized by the generous use of blood transfusions and fluid replacement. Anaesthetics have also advanced in recent years. The result of all these achievements is that surgeons can today operate on people of very advanced years – age is no longer a serious barrier to replacement operations. So take heart if you have arthritis and won't see sixty, or even seventy, again.

5.
ALTERNATIVE THERAPIES

Today, doctors are no longer looked upon as the founts of all wisdom. If you have failed to respond to traditional medical treatments or have friends who have been treated unsuccessfully, you will probably feel like investigating some of the more unusual remedies, or claimed remedies. Some of the treatments mentioned in this chapter have worked successfully for some people, but in many instances the apparent success may be more truly credited to faith than to the efficacy of the treatment concerned.

Try traditional methods first. But then, if these bring you no relief, test less accepted methods carefully. Many of them are supported by doctors who, even though they may not be able to identify how or why a particular treatment works, have seen patients benefit from it.

Faith is, of course, a major factor in cure or treatment. If you believe sincerely that a particular diet or the wearing of a copper bracelet will help your arthritis, it will probably do so. But what must be faced and never forgotten is that one person's panacea may be another's total waste of time or may, indeed, cause harm.

ACUPUNCTURE

Acupuncture is an ancient Chinese therapeutic system. It involves the skilful placing of needles in certain areas of the body to induce local anaesthesia.

The anaesthetic uses of acupuncture are undeniable. It is over twenty years since an eminent professor of anaesthesia at Oxford University described how, during a visit to China, he had seen many major operations, including a lung removal, carried out under acupuncture. But because acupuncture can provide deep anaesthesia in China does not mean it would work equally effectively over here. The Chinese accept this form of anaesthesia in the knowledge that it has been used in their country for centuries. They know it works and have total confidence that they will feel nothing, whatever the surgeon may do. Westerners may accept the concept but, however open-minded, cannot have a similar traditional faith; niggling doubts are bound to intrude.

Because of its anaesthetic capacity, acupuncture can be used successfully to treat pain, but the effects are only temporary. It is as a pain-killer and nothing more that it is of value to you. It cannot possibly improve the condition of a joint that is physically damaged. Many acupuncturists dispute this. They claim that the insertion of tiny gold or silver needles under the skin at particular points will not only stop pain but will also cure the disease. However, no scientific proof has ever been produced which can support this claim.

If, on the other hand, nothing seems to reduce the pain you are in, you could give acupuncture a try. Even a short respite from pain can be a wonderful morale booster.

OSTEOPATHY

Today osteopaths and chiropractors are accepted, respected and used by the medical profession; indeed, many doctors take up these disciplines themselves. Doctors will also refer their patients to these therapists for a variety of ailments.

Osteopaths believe that a large number of diseases are due to the derangement of parts of the skeleton and should therefore be treated by manipulation, returning the wayward joints and bones to their intended sites and strengthening and supporting the muscles controlling them. (The chiropractor has a similar creed but concentrates on the spine.)

Many rheumatic conditions have their source in mechanical malfunction and so it seems logical in these cases to try and get the joints functioning again by manipulating them. However, if your bones or joints are actually damaged, no amount of manipulation or massage can restore them to their former state; ostopathy does not provide a *cure*.

Osteopathy is far more likely to be successful if you have osteoarthritis. If you suffer from rheumatoid arthritis your tissues may be inflamed and any unnecessary movement or manipulation may cause harm rather than benefit.

The spine is a most intricate structure, with many delicate bones and joints. When a rheumatic complaint is diagnosed as the cause of pain, manipulation and/or massage may bring almost miraculous relief. However, in a few cases such treatment can cause damage. So do seek advice from your doctor before trying such treatment, whether from an osteopath or a chiropractor.

Osteopathic treatment for arthritis

Osteopaths treat osteoarthritic patients particularly gently. The state of the bones means that manipulation must be minimal, as flaking or crumbling can easily occur, especially in elderly people. Mobilization of the soft tissues – ligaments and muscles – and of the affected joint by passive movements carried out by the osteopath can both improve the quality of life and allow more freedom of movement with a substantial reduction in pain. Soft tissue mobilization is a pleasant and gentle treatment. The osteopath uses the fingers and palm of his or her hand to locate the origins and insertions of muscles, then helps to release uneven contractions by lifting and manipulating the belly – the middle – of the muscle to encourage circulation and drainage of fluids from the tissue. Muscles are elastic and respond well to this treatment. There are, however, degrees of elasticity; tired or under-used muscles need a lot of encouragement. Much depends on which joints are involved. Weight-bearing joints are more difficult to treat than the upper limbs, but even so, if the condition has not gone too far, it is possible even with hip joints to stabilize the condition and effect some improvement with mobilization and exercises.

An osteopath will help you to re-educate your body and re-align your posture. This will enable more of your muscles to play a part in movements, and so take the load off the affected joint, thereby giving it a chance to rest and, in some cases, to regenerate.

Some osteopaths use seaweed treatments as an adjunct to their normal treatment. Seaweed packs applied to the body and used with heat give relief from pain and are especially useful for elderly patients.

THE MAGIC MUSSEL

All over the world research is going on to find an alternative to drugs as treatment for all forms of arthritis. Today few question the efficacy of drugs in reducing inflammation and deadening pain. But as yet no drug had been developed that can treat arthritis, or indeed any other illness, without having side-effects. Side-effects may not even become apparent until years after the drug has been administered. And when the side-effects do appear, they may be even worse than the condition they were prescribed to treat. This has led to the coining of the word 'iatragenic', meaning disease caused by drugs prescribed to treat another disease.

One of the latest discoveries in the quest for drugless

treatments is the green-lipped mussel, *Perna canalicullus*, from New Zealand. You may well laugh cynically, but in this instance there is now little doubt that the green-lipped mussel does contain an anti-inflammatory compound, which effectively treats arthritis. It was initially tested on rats in a fully authenticated trial conducted by doctors at the

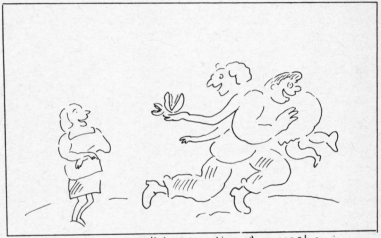

I don't know about this green lipped mussel curing his arthritis but it's certainly made him a lot more passionate

Department of Surgery at the School of Medicine at the University of Auckland. Further research since 1974 has substantiated the claims for the mussel's effectiveness.

The mussel is now 'farmed' on an island off Auckland and extracts made from it are bringing relief to thousands. One of its great advantages over drugs is the lack of gastric side-effects, such as are encountered with aspirin-based drugs.

But, as with all other treatments for arthritis, different people react differently to the treatment. Some have found that after a course they have been able to stop taking it and have had no return of their arthritic symptoms. Others have found it necessary to continue the treatment indefinitely, and that as soon as they omit their daily dose the arthritis returns.

THE COPPER BRACELET

Every now and then you meet someone wearing a copper bracelet who claims that it has cured their arthritis. You may also have read advertisements suggesting that

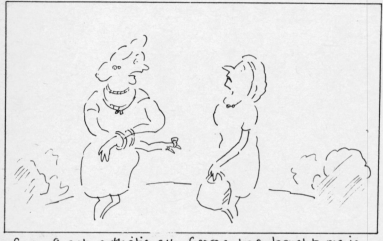

Since I got arthritis all George has bought me is copper bracelets, copper rings, copper necklaces, copper...

wearing such a bracelet is an almost sure-fire cure. Perhaps it is.

The copper intra-uterine device works effectively as a method of contraception. How does it work? No one knows for sure. But it does and its failure rate is only between two and three per cent.

A copper bracelet prevents arthritis. How does it work? No one knows. But *if* it does, the success rate is probably three per cent at most.

ROYAL JELLY

Many claims are made for Royal Jelly, a food gathered,

according to the advertising blurbs, from the beehives of China, 'Where the air is fresh and the flowers plentiful'. Royal Jelly keeps you young and vigorous. It makes you feel one hundred per cent hale and hearty. It relieves all nervous tension. It can bring down blood-pressure and provides resistance to infection. It improves appetite and helps you to sleep. It's been acclaimed for decades as the perfect aphrodisiac and after a course of Royal Jelly a

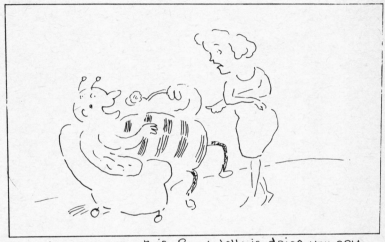

Are you sure this Royal Jelly is doing you any good George?

man becomes capable of fathering a legion and a woman as desirable as Delilah.

If we believe all these assertions, those of us not taking Royal Jelly are undeniably mad. But there is no way of proving or disproving them.

There seems no scientific reason that Royal Jelly should act as a pain-killer, as some of its fans claim. Scientific analysis is said to have identified ten separate vitamins as well as proteins and various elements in it. And that can't be bad! It is, however, extremely expensive, so it is probably only worth trying as a last resort and if you are on good terms with your bank manager!

THALASSOTHERAPIE

In France the national health service will pay up to
seventy per cent of bills for thalassotherapie. That, at
least, should encourage us to approach this very Gallic
treatment with respect. However . . . .

The first centre was opened at Dieppe a century ago,
shortly followed by one at Margate, now abandoned.
Today, in France, this treatment by sea-water and
seaweed is rapidly growing in popularity and is widely
recommended by doctors for patients suffering from
arthritis, among other complaints.

The treatment is based on the theory that sea-water
contains minerals and elements almost identical with
those found in our blood and intra-cellular fluids. The
enthusiastic supporters of thalassotherapie believe that
if the body is immersed in sea-water heated to between
36° and 40° Centigrade, osmosis – percolation – occurs
and the water plus seaweed penetrates the skin and
nourishes the 'sub-dermal' layers.

There's probably little doubt that a period at one of
these extremely well-equipped clinics would work

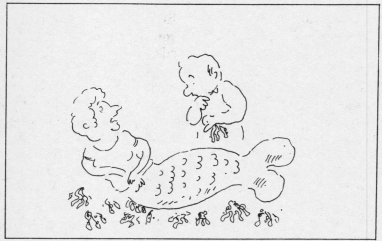

Look Albert if you had been putting seaweed on
your joints and exercising in water for the last five
years you would have turned into a mermaid as well.

wonders for your health. Apart from immersion in sea-water there are special baths, delightfully dubbed *Les bains aesthetic*, rather like jacuzzis, which stimulate every inch of the body. Seaweed packs all over and regular skilful massage could only leave you feeling pampered and purring with contentment. The sense of general well-being can help you to withstand pain better. But the osmosis claims are harder to believe. If liquids could so easily penetrate our skins, we'd become water-logged every time we took a bath or went for a swim.

THE TROGLODYTE'S DIET

This 'cure' for arthritis demands that you completely rethink your eating habits. You begin with a full day's fasting, taking only water. Then gradually you introduce raw fruit and vegetables, raw liver and sea food. You are advised to take cod liver oil daily and must eschew forever any of those foods most of us find most appetising or convenient. No bread, toast, biscuits, pies, spaghetti; in fact, no products that use flour.

No tea, coffee, cocoa, liquor, wine or fizzies.

No sugar in anything.

No foods adulterated with additives, which rules out most tinned foods and requires you to make a careful study of all the labels on the goods you're considering buying.

Of course, such spartan diet demands a will of iron, even though Dr Campbell, who devised it, suggests this isn't so. Indeed, he suggests that we must condition our subconscious computers so that refusal is a reflex action, which doesn't require any exercise of will-power. In his book, *A Home Cure for Arthritis*, he tells us how to relax and to make use of visualization – imagining ourselves when on his diet to be hale, healthy and hopeful, and then when breaking the rules, to be ailing, aged and anxious. Dr Campbell reminds us of the acknowledged dangers of the side-effects of taking drugs and is depressingly convinced that there are no drugs to cure arthritis and that there is little likelihood that any will ever be discovered.

No doubt a friendless person without any social engagements and with a taste for severe self-discipline could manage this regime, which would almost certainly relieve at least some of the symptoms of arthritis, and in some instances might even cure it. But no diet, even this most spartan one, can effect a cure when a joint has sustained actual damage. In cases where the sufferer's life is literally not worth living, the diet might well prove helpful. But most of us will probably say: 'Life's just too short'.

SPAS

Visiting Bath or Leamington, Buxton or Harrogate to take the waters was an accepted part of treatment for rheumatic diseases in the days of our great-grandparents . . . so long as they were fortunate enough to be born into the moneyed classes. Certainly this is a form of treatment with a long history. We know the Romans had water centres which were used for treating many ailments.

There is little doubt that extravagant medical claims have been made for many spas. But once again, the contentment resulting from bathing and the faith that the waters are doing good, will have a beneficial effect on most of us − if we can afford it.

This form of self-indulgence will do little harm, but it's unlikely to do you much good either.

6.
LIVING WITH ARTHRITIS

Arthritis can make even the simplest movement difficult.
Actions that the hale and hearty carry out almost as reflex
movements can becomes real labours of Hercules. Not
only can turning off a tap or turning on a switch be painful
but when your fingers are deformed, these most simple
of tasks can become ordeals.

During acute periods, when, perhaps, surgery has been
the only solution, you will have the support of the doctors,
nurses and therapists fighting to improve the quality of
your life, to make you less handicapped and more able
to cope. But when the fight has been won and you are
ready to go home you are on your own. The therapists
– physio and occupational – will advise and support you,
but they cannot be there all the time. Once back at home
you have to cope whether you like it or not.

Starting up again is a real test of one's resources, both
physical and mental. The nervous strain can be
considerable and nothing can destroy confidence quicker
than frustration. However hard you try, it is difficult to
prevent yourself sometimes thinking: 'I used to do this
so easily, but now . . .'

GENERAL PRINCIPLES

As you will have realized by now, the best thing to do if you have arthritis is to follow the treatment prescribed, accept your condition and try to be objective about it. It is essential to take a cool look at your limitations. What *can* you do? What *can't* you do? Then, having mentally drawn up your balance sheet, it will be easier to make certain that you are using your remaining capabilities to the full and finding ways of dealing with those tasks that are no longer within your range.

This means planning. It means planning not only your home, but also your daily regime and the use you make of your body. There's little use having the most sophisticated machine in the world — your body (even if it does now suffer from arthritis), if you don't keep it running as efficiently as possible. This means keeping your muscles tuned up and your joints working to their full range.

It also means making sure that you are not putting unnecessary strain on your physical resources because your home does not allow for the fact that your are no longer as fit as you were. The dramatist, when plotting an actor's moves, will make sure that the channels of entrance and exit will be free of furniture and props that might get in the way. View your home in the same way. Make sure you can pass freely from one room to another without a piece of furniture, which could easily be sited elsewhere, getting in the way.

Apply the same principle to the various things that you have to do each day. Before you start anything first work out what you will want and where the tools or instruments are likely to be and in what order you'll need them. Make sure those things you'll want most frequently are nearest to hand. Too much reaching up and down not only wastes time but places unnecessary stress on your joints. When you've marshalled your thoughts and your implements, it's the time to take action and only then.

Always buy lightweight equipment, whether it be a frying pan, a trowel for the garden or a fitting for the shower in the bath. The difference may not seem much when you're weighing one against the other in a shop, but in daily use a few ounces can make a hell of a difference, and it is essential to conserve your strength all the time. Compare designs too and don't hesitate to ask if there's anything new on the market. If your hands are gnarled like mine, then look for solid, heavy handles to cups and crockery, kitchen implements and so on. Choose handles which won't require you to worry about their fragility.

Try, too, whenever possible, to avoid putting strain on your smaller joints, particularly your wrists and fingers. Use your larger joints more. Once you stop to think about it, you'll be amazed just how many things you can carry on your forearm rather than in your fingers. And, when going shopping, use a bag that you can carry over your shoulder. This will reduce the strain on your arms and hands.

And if you do succumb to temptation – and you probably will occasionally – and try to move something which you know is really beyond you, at least put your whole weight behind it: use your shoulders and not your arms. And never, ever, use one hand if you can use both. That, indeed, is probably the maxim that best summarizes successful living with arthritis: spread the load. Spend a little time in those early days training yourself to think in this way and it will soon become so automatic that you won't even realize you are thinking like this.

LOOKING AFTER YOURSELF

With the reservations mentioned earlier in the book, you should take exercise regularly, but always within your capacity. If you do not exercise a muscle or joint it will lose strength and mobility and will eventually atrophy, wasting away altogether.

Exercising just for the sake of exercising can be

extremely boring, which increases the temptation not to do it! So, if you can, combine exercising with other pastimes or hobbies. Swimming is one obvious, and very beneficial, example. Walking, too, is good, and if you can walk you can derive pleasure from the scenery, from meeting friends or from looking at paintings while keeping your body in form. Walking, swimming and exercises are not only good for the direct symptoms of arthritis, but also for your general health, improving your heart function, blood circulation and lung capacity. It also defers deterioration of the arteries. And, what is more, there is a tremendous sense of achievement when, after weeks of only being able to manage a few widths of the swimming-pool, you swim a length without stopping.

If exercises are the most convenient way for you to keep fit, make a regular routine of them, doing them at the same time and in the same place each day. Make sure that you gradually extend your range of movement without over-taxing your muscles and joints. Many people find music extremely helpful as it reduces boredom. But don't exercise to anything over-fast or over-rhythmical. Trying to keep in time may result in tying yourself into a knot! At all events be consistent and stick to your plans.

Never forget that pain is the body's warning system. If you suddenly start suffering spasms of pain after exercising, there is a reason. Muscles and joints which should be gently nudged into greater use are liable to strain when they are catapulted into action. There is nothing clever or heroic in trying to cross the pain barrier – leave that to the masochists and professional athletes!

Tension on muscles certainly aggravates aches and pains. So it's not only important to exercise, but also to relax. Just as you set aside periods for exercising, you should also set aside periods for relaxation. It need not be long. Half an hour at a time is quite enough. Make yourself really comfortable. Loosen your clothes and then

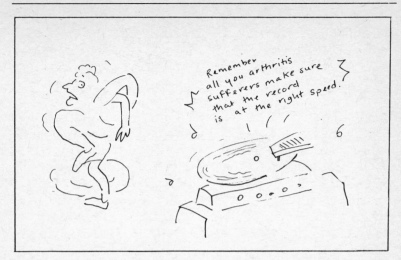

make a conscious effort to relax. It's remarkable how effectively slow, deep breathing can lower tension.

Remember this in those early morning hours when even small problems seem insoluble. Relax and breathe deeply. They will soon return to their right proportions. Think about the various parts of your anatomy and consciously relax each part in turn as you do so. Begin with your toes and concentrate on each one in turn, before starting on the toes of your other foot. Then each foot, each ankle, shin, calf and so on. You'll be amazed how refreshed you feel by the time you've reached your scalp. In fact you may not even reach it, because this relaxation technique is also a good sleep inducer!

Taking care of your appearance is another very important part of looking after yourself– knowing one looks a mess is one of the most efficient ways there is of lowering one's spirits and under-mining self-confidence.

Few of us are fortunate enough to be able to replace our entire wardrobe at one go, and though some of your clothes will prove awkward to get into and fasten, there are plenty of gadgets to help with the problem: aids to help you put on socks and tights without bending, hooks to do up buttons, others to help with zips, and so on. Once you start asking and looking around, you'll be surprised at how many things there are to help you.

When the time comes for new clothes you'll probably find that you view them in a totally different way. However lovely a particular dress may be, if you're exhausted by the time you've managed to get it on, you'll never really be able to enjoy wearing it. Don't choose anything too figure-hugging, particularly if the fastening is at the back. Think before you buy of how you are going to get the clothes on and off. And keeping warm out of doors in winter no longer means heavy bulky coats. Light-weight quilted coats of synthetic fibres have seen to that.

Shoes, too, can be a problem, especially if you have been used to wearing ones that are in keeping with current fashions. It goes without saying that low-heeled styles are the best, but this need not automatically mean the end of a stylish appearance (unless, of course, you want it that way – but that's up to you!). With the interest in general health and sporting leisure activities, there is a very wide range of stylish training shoes around – many never intended to pound around a track or dash about a court – that give your feet support, have velcro fastenings if your fingers can no longer deal with laces, and look smashing with the many ranges of leisure, tracksuit-type wear available in the shops. These clothes also, incidentally, have the merits of being loose, light and warm.

Slippers may seem very tempting if your feet are very painful, but they are not a good idea as they do not give your feet any support. Wear them when you are sitting down, but once you have to get up and start moving around change into shoes. Remember that your feet and ankles take the whole weight of your body, so need all the help and support you can give them, and that comes best from properly fitting shoes.

Of course, if you are wealthy or have particular problems with your feet, the best solution is to have your shoes made for you.

Hair that looks nice is also a very important factor in keeping one's morale high. Painful arms and hands may make it harder for you to continue doing your hair yourself. Discuss the problem with your hairdresser, who will probably be able to advise on a style that will require very little maintenance to keep it looking nice. A well-cut style keeps its shape and looks good for many months, but if you feel that you need to have your hair trimmed more often, now you can't look after it as you used to, don't forget that many hairdressers have reduced charges for pensioners and the disabled and also run hairdressing schools for their trainees. These schools always need guinea-pigs (models is the polite term) and the charges are minimal or non-existent. As the trainees cut and style under the eagle-eye of a senior member of staff you are unlikely to end up looking a freak! And hair washing at home will be much easier if you do it under the shower (see page 90).

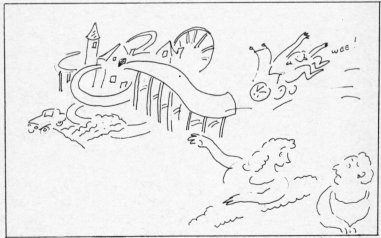

When he said he'd have to make house alterations because of his arthritis I never dreamed he'd go this far.

REPLANNING YOUR HOME

One of the most important things you can do to make

living with arthritis easier is to spend time having a good hard look at you home. Most of us have homes that have grown like Topsy. Bits and pieces of furniture and knick-knacks have been brought in higgledy-piggledy. Perhaps that cupboard was shifted to make way for the television set; that cabinet for a stool. Couldn't that chair, which you always have to walk round, be moved elsewhere?

If you have arthritis you are probably going to have to spend long periods at home, so examine your room(s) critically. What do you do in the sitting-room most often? What is your route across the room when you are going to make tea? You will have to get out of your chair to answer the door, so would it be worth moving it to the other side of the television set? Imagine your home empty and then rearrange the furniture with the knowledge your examination has given you into your habits – something you've probably never given any thought to before!

It may well be worth inviting the occupational therapist round to give you professional advice. Certainly when everything is in place it always helps to have a fresh, objective opinion on the matter. The therapist will also be able to advise you where to position wall supports if they are necessary, and will also be able to suggest what other gadgets might make your life easier.

Entrances and stairs

There are so many small, finicky things that cause those of us with arthritis delay and frustration. And trying to get keys into locks with arthritic fingers must come high in the frustration-inducing league! If you know that you have trouble with this and are not too confident about being steady on your feet, or the step outside your front door is too narrow to balance on with your stick, have a grab-handle or rail fixed so that you can steady yourself with that while doing battle with the door keys. Don't forget, however, that there are special gadgets to ease this problem. Ask your occupational therapist about them, don't feel too shy or too proud – after all what's the point of hanging about on a cold doorstep fumbling with keys if you can be indoors with the kettle on for a hot drink quicker by using a gadget?

If you have to deal with stairs, either to get to your front door, or inside your home, do make sure you have strong handrails fixed. If you have one hand or arm stronger than the other, do not rely on the bannisters because unless you go up and down stairs sideways (and who wants to do that?) you will have to support yourself with your weak hand or arm on either the ascent or descent. And its a fact of life that if you're slightly nervous about stumbling or falling, you are much more likely to do so!

There are special electrically-driven chairs that can be fixed to the bannisters and so carry you upstairs without the necessity of climbing the stairs. Sadly, it goes without saying that useful though these are, they are enormously expensive and so beyond the pockets of most of us.

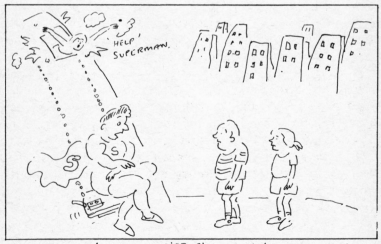

Since my joints got stiff I've started using a chair lift.

Living rooms

If you are going to have to spend more time at home than usual, your living room is likely to be even more important to you than it was before, and the most important item in it will be your chair. It is difficult to over-estimate the importance of this piece of furniture and the effect it will have on the quality (or otherwise) of your life. When assessing the suitability of a chair for your needs, there are certain basic principles to bear in mind.

First of all is safety. The chair must stand firmly on the ground without a hint of a wobble. It may be convenient for cleaning to have castors on each of the legs so it can be shifted at a touch when hoovering, but that's a small asset if the chair shoots away just as you're lowering yourself into it. For maximum stability the front legs should be straight and at a right angle to the floor, perfectly perpendicular in fact, so that when you get up out of the chair, your thrust is directly downwards with the weight going through the chair's legs to the floor. The back legs can be curved if you prefer, but should be angled backwards so as to meet directly the backward thrust of your body's weight as you sit down in the chair. This will preclude any danger of the chair tipping over backwards.

The chairarms should be firm and either unpadded or with very little padding. If your hands are arthritic you need to be able to grip the arms as firmly as possible, and as you push downwards to get up the feeling of firm resistance to the direction of your movement is very reassuring.

The backs should be shaped to give maximum support to your spine; the whole length and not just one section. The seat should be at a height to allow you to place your feet firmly on the floor while sitting comfortably. A too wide chair, though looking stylish, is unlikely to provide as much support for your back and sides as a narrower one.

When relaxing it is important that your neck is

supported. This is where many otherwise excellent chairs fail. The best chairs have canopies over the back which end in a weight. This not only keeps the canopy straight and uncreased, but allows easy adjustment of the pillow-like neck pad inside its folds. Failing this, be sure there is a neck-rest which is not only sufficiently stuffed and well shaped, but can be fixed in different positions. You won't always want to sit in exactly the same way, sometimes you will want to be more upright and at other times to slump more – whatever your physiotherapist might say!

Look at your chairs bearing these principles in mind. Do you have any that meet these criteria, apart, perhaps, from the head-rest? If you have, make sure that it becomes the chair that you use whenever you sit down for any length of time. If you haven't, use the one that comes nearest to fulfilling the criteria and, if at all possible, start to save for one that really fulfils your needs – it is not an extravagance or an indulgence, but rather a vital necessity.

When you go out to buy chair for yourself, you'll probably be very surprised just how many special chairs there are on the market. If you're rich, or have just had a sudden windfall, go for the Jefferson Chair. This, as the name suggests, was designed by the President of the United States, Thomas Jefferson. By training an architect and designer, Jefferson conceived the idea that we are at our most efficient when we are relaxed. This was a revolutionary idea in the early 19th century, when it was widely believed that for anything to be good for you it must look ugly or taste nasty. The modern Jefferson Chair celebrates the President's invention. It is a haven of sheer luxury. Every section of it can be exactly adjusted to your size and shape, however peculiar. It supports every vertebra and provides rests for your limbs. If you're working, there's a tray which carries your typewriter, sewing things or book. Another smaller tray is at your elbow for your cup of tea or gin and tonic. There is an attachment for your computer. Spotlights from various angles illuminate whatever you are doing. Once installed in the Jefferson Chair you want to stay there . . . if only it weren't for the need to eat or the calls of nature. Marvellous! But very, very costly.

More within the range of most of us are a whole variety of chairs especially designed for those with arthritis or posture difficulties. Some are made to measure and these are not nearly so expensive as you might imagine. It is well worth finding out approximate costs before you reject the idea out of hand. Sadly, many chairs excellent in every other way are not attractive and seem to smack of the surgery. Designers are now much more aware of this fact and are today giving careful thought to appearance – after all our spirits need just as much cosseting as our bodies.

Second-hand chairs are another possibility and can be excellent value if chosen to suit your needs, following the principles outlined on pages 84 to 85. Ask your physiotherapist for an opinion if you are in any doubt. Your local social services might know of any second-hand chairs that are available, though putting an advertisement in a local shop or newspaper is also worth trying.

Having bought your chair, don't skimp on the covering if it has one. You are going to use it in your home, and though in some ways it may be a surgical aid, why remind yourself and everyone else of that each time you look at the chair?

Before you settle down comfortably in your chair, make sure that everything you are going to need is within easy reach. And, if you haven't got one already, what about getting a remote control for your television set?

Bedrooms
Most of us spend more time in every forty-eight hours in our beds than anywhere else, and many of us will have slept in the same beds for years even though they have been sagging for decades. They're our beds and we accept them as such. This is extremely short-sighted. A sagging

bed means unnatural strains on spine and limbs and
waking up in the morning with aches and pains or even
cramps. Today beds can cost thousands or even a few
pounds, so it's worth shopping around. There are, of
course, special orthopaedic beds, which may sadly be
beyond our pockets. But plain wooden planks placed
under a mattress can transform an ordinary bed into a
very good imitation of an orthopaedic one, if you don't
want to buy a new one. A firm mattress is absolutely
essential.

Having dealt with your bed and its mattress, what
about its height? Can you get in and out of it easily? Make
sure your bed is at the right height for *you* even if it means
chopping a few inches off the legs.

If getting in and out is impossible without help, there
are a variety of hoists available. Once again turn to your
occupational therapist who will be able to judge where
and what help you need and advise on where hoists can
be bought. Ask too, if you can get a grant towards the
cost. Funds are available, in certain circumstances, for
this purpose.

Having settled the question of your bed and adapted
it to your present needs, or bought a new one, think about
what you put on it. If you've been using the same bed
for years the chances are that you've been using the
bedclothes for equally long. Do consider the advantages
of a duvet if you don't use one. Bedmaking really is
reduced to a minimum – just a twitch or two to plump
up the duvet and get it back in position and your bed
is made. There is no more bending to tuck sheets and
blankets in under the mattress, or the struggle to get
them straight before you even reach that stage! And
putting a fresh duvet cover on isn't difficult because the
duvet itself is light and the opening in the cover is
large.

And what about the position of the bed? Have you
thought about that? If you've always had it in a corner
against a wall, it'll make bedmaking much easier (if you
are sticking to sheets and blankets) to have it away from

the wall so that you won't have to pull it away and then push it back again every day when you make it.

Sex and arthritis

While on the subject of bedrooms it seems appropriate to mention sex. Far too often sex between those who are getting on or are handicapped, is looked upon as a little indecent, or if not indecent, as a little embarrassing. Yet sex is one of the only activities in which the aged or those of limited movement can take part and give each other pleasure without hurt to either and which, most importantly, can transcend chronic pain. Apart from the physical relief, sex can also relieve depression, which is a common companion of constant arthritis aches and pains. Depression frequently leads to irrational and angry outbursts usually directed against those nearest and dearest. Sex provides an outlet for this anger, replacing it with love and affection.

Sex is more important for some people than for others, but however strong or weak our libidos, or however disabled we are by arthritis, most of us can manage to make love so long as we are not afraid or too embarrassed

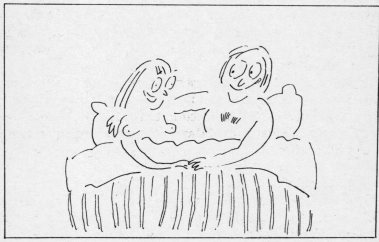

With all these new positions we have to find I wish we'd got arthritis earlier!

to use imagination and ingenuity.

What has to be appreciated from the outset is that spontaneity may have to be jettisoned. Sex for the elderly or disabled often involves careful planning.

A warm bath may well help to relax stiff or over-taxed muscles. Gentle pre-sex exercises or even taking pain-killers in anticipation may solve what formerly appeared to be insoluble problems. For many couples the loss of spontaneity may be compensated for by the sense of togetherness and anticipation involved in the planning.

If you or your partner become limited in movement, you may both feel unable to solve all the problems, whether physical or psychological. There are, however, highly qualified counsellors, who have heard similar stories many times. They can advise and reassure those who have the initiative to seek their advice. They will explain that, in all but very special circumstances, sex is not only possible but need have no unpleasant after-effects.

If, however, you or your partner have recently had a hip-replacement operation sex is *not* advisable. Intercourse less than a month afterwards might well result in dislocation. And it's difficult to think of the position of your legs when you're making love. Even when full intercourse is out of the question, this need not mean celibacy. Oral sex or mutual masturbation involves no risk of dislocation.

The replacement by surgery of joints can in many cases enable patients to have intercourse even after years of enforced celibacy. But the couple who really want to give each other pleasure will always find a way of overcoming the difficulties.

Bathrooms
The bathroom can be a chamber of horrors for anyone disabled. Expert advice is vital to avoid falling or hurting yourself getting in and out of the bath or using the toilet.

Solving the problem of using the toilet isn't too difficult.

The seat must be at the right height and many manufacturers produce attachments which can be clipped onto the existing seat, thus raising it to the required height.

Bathing invariably involves the risk of slipping. It is most important that handrails should be sited in exactly the right place on the walls as well as the bath sides. It is only too easy to grab for support and begin to panic when you don't immediately find the rail under your fingers. To prevent slipping, the bottom of the bath should not be smooth and there are many non-slip materials available, some of which are prettily patterned, to prevent the bath bottom becoming an ice-rink.

The bath mat should not be the ordinary variety which is liable to send you skidding the moment you put your foot on it. It should be of an adhering nature, or have suckers to anchor it to the floor. If it is difficult for you to lie flat in the bath, there are stools especially designed so that you can sit in the water. Unfortunately, most of them have a somewhat clinical appearance. Steps are also available to help you get into the bath when the sides are too high.

If you are very disabled, you will probably find a hoist necessary to help you get in and out of the bath. Ask the advice of your occupational therapist about the type that is best for you, and also if you are eligible for a grant towards the cost of buying and installing the hoist.

However, from the point of view of safety, showers have a very real advantage over baths, because they do away with the problem of having to lower yourself perilously into the bath and dragging yourself out afterwards.

Showers come in all shapes and sizes varying from the hand-held jet attached by rubber tubing to the bath taps, to a luxurious cubicle designed by experts so it occupies no more space than the average-sized bath.

Showering in one of these cubicles is opulence itself, but sadly can only be indulged in by the very rich. Subdued lighting and heat radiate down on you from above. Three separate nozzles – at head, navel and ankle

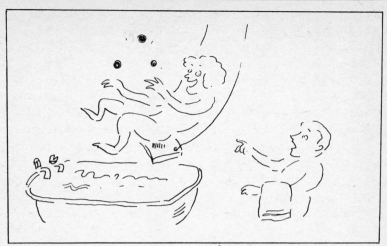

This is supposed to be a hoist for the bath not a circus trapeze.

level – direct their jets to every part of your body without demanding any exertion except switching a button. The seat is adjustable so you can stand or sit, whichever takes your fancy. Hot towels can be drawn into the cubicle from the heated airing cupboard outside. There are vertical and horizontal safety rails with a beautifully designed soap dish on the horizontal rail so that it is always close to the portion of your anatomy you're washing at that moment. The floor is patterned with non-slip material and the glass door opens at a touch should you feel suddenly claustrophobic. This is for you . . . if you've already made your fortune!

For the rest of us, with our more modest means, there is such a wide choice of showers that some will be within everyone's budget. For a moderate outlay you can have a most efficient shower fitted for use while you are standing in the bath. Showering like this still leaves you with the problems of having to clamber in and out of the bath, but at least you will not have to lower yourself in and out of the water, with all the problems and discomfort caused by these manoeuvres. Ideally, it is best to have a shower as a separate unit into which you can step with the minimum of difficulty. There are a number of these units on the market, and some can even go in the bedroom if the bathroom is not big enough.

Kitchens

If you have arthritis the problems posed by the kitchen and all the activities that go on in it may appear very daunting. But they are not nearly as intractable as they may at first seem. It is very important to take a good hard look at how you use the kitchen, thinking about the moves you routinely make when preparing food, cooking and washing up afterwards. Then ask yourself if you could do the same things in another way, a way that reduces the number of times you have to cross the kitchen, for example. Be objective. This is an exercise to help you conserve your energy, not a criticism of the way you always did things before.

Many people with arthritis find it easier to sit down to cook, so bear this in mind when deciding on the position and height of the oven, sink(s) and the preparation area. (In the kitchen as elsewhere in your home, all electric plugs, sockets and switches should be sited at convenient places and heights to reduce the risk of falling or stumbling as you bend or stretch to reach them.)

It is most important we should relax as often as possible, so our kitchens should be planned with this in mind and care should be taken to eliminate any unnecessary movements. If preparation boards, serving, cooking and washing up areas can be sited around your chair so you don't have to get up and sit down again to work at them, so much to the good.

Make sure, too, that your working area is properly lit, and do make sure that all your switches are large enough for you – here and in the other rooms.

It is also worth taking time to consider how best to store your pots and pans so you do not have to bend or stretch every time you need one. For the lighter utensils it is usually more convenient to have hooks on which to hang them. You cannot have too many hooks in the kitchen.

There are always things you need to have handy. And despite the nuisance of cleaning them, plenty of shelves means room for all those spices, herbs and so on which always seem to gather round you if you are a keen cook.

Drawers should be easily opened and capacious, there is little worse than having to pull and tug at a drawer when you're sitting down and have little purchase. Rails for safety should be attached wherever possible. It gives reassurance. And if you use a stick, choose one with a crooked top and not a flat handle, you'll find it easier to hook onto one of your safety rails rather than trying to lean it up against the furniture with the ever present risk of it falling and you having to decide how to pick it up again.

The washing-up area also deserves special consideration. Washing up is an unrewarding chore at the best of times. So make the effort to ensure it takes as little of your time as possible. Ideally, if there is enough space, have two sinks, one for washing and one for rinsing. The plate rack should be close enough to the rinsing sink so that you don't have to stand up to load it. Of course a washing machine simplifies all this . . . but again cost raises its ugly head. However, if you can afford one, don't forget to have it put at a convenient level. No good saving washing time if you've got to rick your back every time you load or unload it.

Having replanned your kitchen have a look at the range of gadgets available and designed especially for people with deformed hands: extensions to taps, rocking kettles to avoid scalding yourself when making tea, vegetable scrapers which remove skin from fruit and veg without doing the same to your hands, scoopers for eating, drinking vessels and non-spill plates. Again your occupational therapist who will advise you on which of these utensils is necessary and which are luxuries in which you should only indulge when you've got spare cash.

Think, too, about the various actions you use, probably

automatically, in cooking. Most of us lift things up quite unnecessarily. On your cooker, for example, it may be possible to slide the pans from one ring to another. But if you do have to lift a pan, try to use the palm of your hand rather than your fingers, and both hands instead of one. Picking up a mug, for instance, can, if it is not too hot, be done with the palm of both hands rather than picking it up with a finger round the handle.

And have you ever thought about just how heavy water can be? Try putting your prepared vegetables into a dry saucepan and then take it to the tap, rather than carry a saucepan of water about unnecessarily. For the same reason, you may well find it helpful to buy one or two double-handed saucepans, so that each hand and arm takes part of the weight. This, in fact, is easier than trying to carry a conventional, single-handled saucepan with both hands.

General housework
Try to do as many chores as possible sitting down. It is remarkable how much you can do from a chair if you use a little ingenuity. You can, for instance, iron quite effectively sitting down. Most ironing boards are adjustable in height, so you can fix yours to suit the height of your chair. A travelling iron, too, will reduce the strain on your wrist and elbow. And, quite as much to the point, ask yourself if what you are about to iron *really* needs it. Answer the question honestly, and you may well save yourself a lot of unnecessary strain and tiredness.

Use tap turners wherever you have taps, they make turning taps on and off so very much easier. When wringing out wet clothes or towels if you don't have a washing machine to do it for you, wrap them around a tap and twist them in one direction using both hands. Doing it this way doesn't put nearly so much strain on the wrists and fingers as twisting one hand against the other.

Try not to fill your washing machine to its full capacity as this will reduce the amount of bending you have to do when loading and unloading it, although this is admittedly a rather extravagant way to use it. Many washing machines have special half-load programmes. If yours has one, use it rather than the full load. And when the times comes to replace your old machine, look out for one with this facility.

RETHINKING YOUR LEISURE

The principles which applied to the rethinking and replanning of your home can also be applied to other areas of your life, not least your leisure activities. 'Friends' may urge you to give up some activity which you've always enjoyed. It may be necessary. It also may *not*. It may be merely a matter of changing your approach or getting mechanical aids to do something which you formerly did without difficulty. And even that is not the whole answer. As well as keeping on with past activities, it is equally important to keep your mind open to new ideas; indeed, whenever possible, embrace new challenges. As well as keeping your body going it will help you avoid sinking into self-pity, an attitude that will lose you friends very quickly.

Of course, it may not be possible to carry on with some of your former activities, but that doesn't mean necessarily abandoning them completely. If you enjoyed acting in amateur dramatics, for example, while there may not be many starring roles for those on sticks or crutches, what about offering your services as stage-manager, prompter, or even as teacher to the newcomers?

You may even be able to help your local sports club as a coach in some sport which you have always enjoyed and played to a reasonable standard, but in which you can no longer take an active part. Ask, find out, the only person who can write you off is you.

If you have a car, you'll be able to find out about the adaptations that will enable you to go on using it comfortably and safely. *And* your parking problems will be virtually over, as you will probably be eligible for concessionary parking facilities.

However, being a passenger in someone else's car can pose problems. If you are the driver you can stop as often as you want to stretch your legs and exercise stiffening muscles and joints, and there's nothing your passengers, if any, can do about it! Not so easy if it is you who are the passenger. But for the sake of everyone, not least you, get into the habit of saying politely, but firmly, before a journey starts that there will be a stop every hour for a brief walk-about to stop your joints seizing up. A hostile reaction will at least tell you who to avoid in future!

The same principle applies when you are visiting friends or anywhere where you are invited to 'take a seat'. Make a point of looking round for the highest chair and

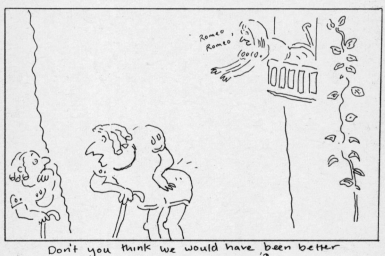

Don't you think we would have been better doing 'The Phantom of the Opera'?

ask for that one. If at first you feel shy about taking this line, a few miserable evenings spent sitting in unsuitable chairs and wondering however you will get out of them, will soon demonstrate the wisdom of the straightforward approach.

Plan your days to husband your resources, examine the ways in which you do things to see if you can save energy, and try doing something before you decide it's impossible and out of the question. You may not be able to do all the things you used to be able to do, but you'll soon find that arthritis need not be a fate worse than death after all.

USEFUL
ADDRESSES

Acupuncture Association and Register
34 Alderney Steet
London SW1
Tel: 01-834 1012

Age Concern
Bernard Sunley House
60 Pitcairn Road
Mitcham
Surrey
Tel: 01-640 5431

Arthritis British Rheumatism Association
6 Grosvenor Crescent
London SW1
Tel: 01-235 0902

Arthritis and Rheumatism Council for Research
41 Eagle Street
London WC1
Tel: 01-405 8572

Association of Carers
Medway House
Balfour Road
Rochester
Kent
Tel: (0634) 813981

Back Pain Association
Grundy House
31/33 Park Road
Teddington
Middlesex
Tel: 01-977 5474/5

British College of Naturopathy and Osteopathy
Fraxer House
6 Netherall Gardens
London NW3
Tel: 01-435 7830

Chartered Society of Physiotherapy
14 Bedford Row
London WC1
Tel: 01-242 1941

Citizens Advice Bureau
(Head Office)
115/123 Pentonville Road
London N1
Tel: 01-833 2181

College of Health
18 Victoria Park Square
London E2
Tel: 01-980 6263

College of Occupational Therapists
1 Needham Road
London W11
Tel: 01-221 6599/6560

Council and Care for the Elderly
131 Middlesex Street
London E1
Tel: 01-621 1624

Health Education Council
78 New Oxford Street
London WC1
Tel: 01-631 0930

Help the Aged
(Head Office)
St James Walk
London EC1
Tel: 01-253 0253

Institute for Complementary Medicine
21 Portland Place
London W1
Tel: 01-636 9543

Intractable Pain Society of Britain
Derby Royal Infirmary
London Road
Derby
Tel: (0332) 47141

National Council for Carers and Elderly Dependants
29 Chilworth Mews
London W2
Tel: 01-262 1451

Osteopathic Medical Association
28 Wimpole Street
London W1
Tel: 01-631 5215

Osteopaths' General Council and Register
1 Suffolk Street
London SW1
Tel: 01-839 2060

Osteopathic Naturopathic College and Clinic
6 Netherhall Gardens
London NW3
Tel: 01-435 7836

Patients' Association
18 Charing Cross Road
London WC2
Tel: 01-240 0671

Pain Relief Foundation
Walton Hospital
Liverpool
Tel: 051-523 1486

Spinal Injuries Association
Yeoman's House
St James' Lane
London N10
Tel: 01-444 9082

FURTHER READING

Arthritis, William Fox (pub: Hale)

Arthritis Another Way (The Magic Mussel), Desmond Zwar (pub: Ideas Unlimited, Australia)

The Arthritis Handbook, Christian Barnard (pub: Michael Joseph)

Arthritis, Julian Freeman (pub: Orbis)

The Arthritis Help Book, Kate Lorig and James Fries (pub: Souvenir)

Bach Flower Therapy, Mechtild Scheffer (pub: Thorsons)

A Doctor's Proven New Home Cure for Arthritis, Giraud W. Campbell (pub: Thorsons)

Essential Rheumatology for Nurses and Therapists, G. S. Panay (pub: Baillière Tindall)

Medicine for Nurses, Arnold Bloom (pub: Churchill Livingstone)

New Hope for the Arthritic, Dr Colin H. Dong and Jane Banks (pub: Granada)

Overcoming Arthritis, Max Warnbrand (pub: Bachman and Turner)

Overcoming Arthritis, Dr Frank Dudley Hart (pub: Martin Dunitz)

Relief from Arthritis, John E. Croft (pub: Thorsons)

Rheumatism and Arthritis, Malcolm Jayson and Alan Dixon (pub: Pan)

Royal Jelly, Irene Steen (pub: Thorsons)

Symptoms, Signs and Syndromes, B. Champney and F. G. Smiddy (pub: Baillière Tindall)

GLOSSARY

Acute – Unlike its general use, in medicine acute has no reference to the severity of pain, but refers to its rapid onset and generally short duration.

Ankylosis – The condition of a joint in which movements are limited by fibrous bands, by malformation or by disease of the bones.

Antigens – Antigens are substances which produce antibodies, nature's forces for fighting invading poisons.

Charcot's joints – Joints where gross arthritis and disruption of the joints are seen in wasting diseases. The result of injury to a joint which has lost the sense of pain and so the disease progresses unheeded.

Chronic – Referring to pain, or disease, of long duration, often with gradual onset.

Corticosteroids – The generic name for the group of hormones with cortisone-like actions.

Herbenden's nodes – A condition affecting the elderly – almost always women. Small swellings appear in the finger-joints, usually those furthest from the wrist. At first soft, in time they become bone.

Lesions – A term originally employed to describe injuries, but now applied to all changes in organs or tissue caused by disease. Disturbance of the structure or function of a part of the body. Can be a wound, abcess, tumour or chemical abnormality.

Prosthesis – An artificial replacement for a part of the body. Can be applied to limb, a false eye or even a set of dentures.

Rheumatism – A general term used to cover a whole group of diseases which mainly manifest themselves in inflammatory or degenerative effects on the fibrous texture of joints, muscle and other parts. Usually any painful disorder not directly owing to infection or injury. It is an ill-defined term as it includes rheumatic fever, rheumatoid arthritis, osteoarthritis, gout and fibrositis.

Steroids – A group of compounds chemically resembling cholesterol. They include the sex hormones, the hormones of the adrenal cortex and the bile acids. Hormones are chemicals manufactured in one organ and then released into the blood stream and so passed to another organ which it activates.

Subacute – Between acute and chronic.

Synovial joints – Joints within the smooth membrane linings *(Synovium)*.

Thoracic joints – Joints within the compartment of the body enclosed by the ribs – the chest.

Trauma – Disorders originating from wounds or injuries.

INDEX

ABOUT THE AUTHOR

TONY VAN DEN BERGH is a distinguished writer and broadcaster in the medical field.

He was interviewer, narrator and researcher on the BBC radio series *Lifelines of Medicine* for nine years. Since 1982, he has been presenter and author of Central Television's *Getting On* series.

He has written many major articles for magazines like *The Listener* and *Arthritis News* and several books on a wide variety of topics – both medical and non-medical.

He lives in North London, and was a founder member of ASM (Action for Smoking and Health).